# Taking Control of Your Nursing Career

## Second Edition

# Taking Control of Your Nursing Career

## Second Edition

*Gail J. Donner, RN, PhD*
*Mary M. Wheeler, RN, MEd*

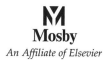

**Mosby**
*An Affiliate of Elsevier*

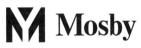 Mosby

An Elsevier Canada Imprint

**National Library of Canada Cataloguing in Publication Data**

Taking control of your nursing career / Gail J. Donner, Mary M. Wheeler, editors. – 2nd ed.

Previously publ. under title: Taking control of your career and your future.
Includes bibliographical references and index.
ISBN 0-920513-49-2

1. Nursing–Vocational guidance.  2. Career development.  I. Donner, Gail J. (Gail Judith) date. II. Wheeler, Mary M.

RT82.T33 2003              610.73'06'9              C2003-903259-0

Acquisitions Editor: Ann Millar
Developmental Editor: Eliza Marciniak
Publishing Services Manager: Deborah L. Vogel
Senior Project Manager: Jodi M. Willard
Design Manager: Mark Bernard


Elsevier Canada
1 Goldthorne Ave., Toronto, ON, Canada M8Z 5S7
Phone: 1-866-896-3331
Fax: 1-866-359-9534


This book was printed in U.S.A.
  2 3 4 5    07 06 05 04

This book is dedicated to our friends and colleagues in the nursing profession whose hard work, commitment, and determination continue to inspire us to believe that nursing really can be a career for life.

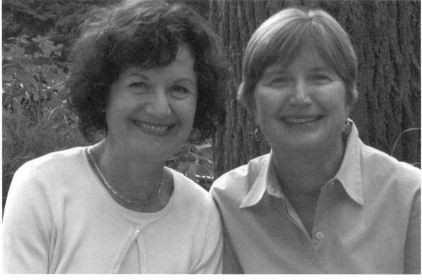

**Gail J. Donner, RN, PhD,** is a Partner in donnerwheeler, Career Development Consultants and Professor Emeritus and former Dean at the Faculty of Nursing, University of Toronto. She has presented numerous papers, seminars, and workshops on a variety of nursing and health care topics. Gail has been active on a number of boards and committees within nursing and in the community at large and has been honoured by several organizations for her contributions. Currently she is a member of the Board of Trustees of the Hospital for Sick Children and is a volunteer for the Toronto Out of the Cold Program and St. Christopher's House. In 2002, Gail received the Ontario Medical Association Centennial Award, which is given to a non-physician for significant contributions to health care in Ontario. In 2001, Gail received the Order of Ontario, the province's highest and most prestigious honour. In 1994 she was named a Woman of Distinction by the YWCA of Metropolitan Toronto and in 1989 was awarded the Registered Nurses Association of Ontario Award of Merit. The new love in Gail's life (after husband, Arthur) is grandson Theodore, with whom she currently spends as much time as possible.

**Mary M. Wheeler, RN, MEd,** has had a varied career that has included positions in practice, management, and education. Before starting her own business, Mary M. Wheeler and Associates, in 1991 and before her partnership with Gail Donner in 1992, Mary worked for the Registered Nurses Association of Ontario. Mary, a certified coach, brings to her practice her expertise and experience in organizational and human resource development and coaching. She also has a special interest in exploring ways in which individuals can use creativity and active reflection to unleash their potential. She divides her time between her home office in Brampton, Ontario and her cottage on the Bruce Peninsula, where she hikes, kayaks, and cycles.

Gail Donner and Mary Wheeler established donnerwheeler in Canada in 1992. Since then, they have worked in Canada, the United States, Europe, and South Africa to build organizational capacity by promoting employee career resilience. Their work includes organizational consulting, onsite and online workshops, individual coaching, publishing, and public speaking on career development. Their five-phase career planning and development model helps nurses to take control of their careers and develop realistic and satisfying plans for the future.

Gail and Mary would be pleased to answer your career planning and development queries. They can be contacted through this text's accompanying website:
*www.elsevier.ca/DonnerWheeler/.*

# CONTRIBUTORS

**Sue Bookey-Bassett, RN, BScN, MEd**
Professional Development Consultant in Nursing,
Oakville, Ontario

**Michelle Cooper, RN, MScN**
President,
Integral Visions Consulting, Inc.,
Ancaster, Ontario;
Associate, donnerwheeler
Brampton, Ontario

**Gail J. Donner, RN, PhD**
Partner, donnerwheeler,
Brampton, Ontario;
Professor Emeritus,
Faculty of Nursing,
University of Toronto,
Toronto, Ontario

**Claire Mallette, RN, MSc, PhD (cand.)**
Chief Nursing Officer, Director of Professional Practice,
Workplace Safety and Insurance Board,
Toronto, Ontario;
PhD candidate,
Faculty of Nursing,
University of Toronto,
Toronto, Ontario

**Linda McGillis Hall, RN, MSc, PhD**
Assistant Professor,
Faculty of Nursing,
University of Toronto,
Totonto, Ontario;
New Investigator,
Canadian Institutes of Health Research,
Ottawa, Ontario;
Co-Investigator,
Nursing Effectiveness, Utilization, and Outcomes Research Unit,
Toronto, Ontario;
Associate, donnerwheeler,
Brampton, Ontario

**Janice Waddell, RN, MA, PhD**
Associate Professor, Associate Director,
School of Nursing,
Ryerson University,
Toronto, Ontario;
Associate, donnerwheeler,
Brampton, Ontario

**Mary M. Wheeler, RN, MEd**
Partner, donnerwheeler,
Brampton, Ontario

**Margot Young, MA, CHRP**
President, Margot Young & Associates Ltd.,
Toronto, Ontario

## REVIEWERS

**Lynda Atack**
Centennial College,
Toronto, Ontario

**Marilyn Beaton**
Memorial University of Newfoundland,
St John's, Newfoundland and Labrador

**Marianne W. Lamb**
Queen's University,
Kingston, Ontario

**Gail Tomblin Murphy**
Dalhousie University,
Halifax, Nova Scotia

**Elizabeth Polakoff**
Red River College,
Winnipeg, Manitoba

**Darlene Steven**
Lakehead University,
Thunder Bay, Ontario

## ACKNOWLEDGEMENTS

As with the first edition, this second edition of *Taking Control of Your Nursing Career* is the result of the work of a number of people. Quite simply, the book and we are better for their contributions. Thanks to chapter authors Linda McGillis Hall, Claire Mallette, Sue Bookey-Bassett, Janice Waddell, Michelle Cooper, and Margot Young for their enthusiasm, their good humour, and their willingness to share their knowledge and experience. Thanks also to Indra Nunner and Manuel Gitterman of aLight, Toronto, Ontario, who designed the wonderful graphic for our model.

In addition, we want to acknowledge the Canadian Nurses Association—publisher of the first edition—and our colleagues who participated as chapter authors in the first edition for helping us bring our work to the nursing community.

Thanks also to Nadia Gulezko for her research and administrative support and to Arthur Reinstein for his assistance with the legal work. To the reviewers of the first draft of this edition of the book, whose contributions to the final version were invaluable—thank you, colleagues.

Special recognition goes to Ann Millar, Acquisitions Editor at Elsevier Canada, who saw the possibilities in our work and whose continuing support and encouragement has been very important to us. Eliza Marciniak acted as Developmental Editor; thank you, Eliza. Jodi Willard was an excellent Project Manager—her expertise and patience are very much appreciated. We also want to thank the rest of the Elsevier team—designers, production people, and everyone else involved in helping us put our best words forward.

Finally, in this project and throughout our careers, we have benefited from the unconditional support and encouragement of our families. They continue to inspire us to be and do more, and for this they have our gratitude and love.

*Gail J. Donner*
*Mary M. Wheeler*

# FOREWORD

Gail Donner and Mary Wheeler have given nursing a wonderful gift. Readers will like the tone of *Taking Control of Your Nursing Career* as well as the essential information for planning and getting the most out of your nursing career at each stage of career development.

Nursing offers a meaningful and rewarding career—being with people in some of their most significant life passages. Not many people can plan a career in which they know they will have a direct hand in people's lives in critical situations and in times of growth and crisis. Nursing offers these options. However, nursing has multiple career trajectories and exists in a complex health care environment with numerous opportunities. Nurses are shown how to assess global and local trends in order to make the most of the opportunities and to assess how they can tailor their career plans to the emerging and complex changes in society and health care. This book explodes the myth of single-track careers in nursing and provides useful tools to the individual nurse in making the most of these societal and health care changes.

The authors provide a wonderful plan for self-reflection. Scanning the immediate environment and larger context is a monitoring and assessment skill that nurses use in clinical practice. In this book, the reader is taught how to use these skills for optimum career planning and development. The authors point out the long and varied career options offered in nursing. To make the most of the wide range of options in nursing, it is essential to gain experiential wisdom in practice and to learn to keep a watchful eye on the opportunities available.

Many career stalls and failures can be accounted for by not knowing one's own values, strengths, and limitations. In the phase of the model "Completing Your Self-Assessment and Reality Check," the authors coach nurses on how to create a realistic assessment of strengths and areas for growth. This requires not only astute self-assessment but also honest appraisals from those who work closely with you.

Creating a career vision is essential to seeing and seizing opportunities. Donner and Wheeler provide readers with the tools for envisioning and actualizing meaningful and rewarding work. Helping nurses see the possibilities and then articulate what they want and how they can make a difference is critical to ensuring a positive future for nurses and for nursing. However, they don't stop with the dream; rather Donner and Wheeler go on to provide some very practical planning strategies for transforming those visions into reality. The self-marketing strategies provide all the essential tools for presenting oneself in complex health care arenas.

In the second part of the book, *Taking Control of Your Nursing Career* provides guidance to nurses at all stages of career development. It will allow the nursing student to imagine the options available over a career lifetime, will help mid-career nurses find meaning in nursing again, and will provide assistance for nurses contemplating retirement. Readers will find it a resource to which they can return many times.

I enthusiastically endorse this book for nurses at each step in making the most of the wonderful opportunities to develop themselves as nurses and human beings while contributing to society through nursing.

*Patricia Benner, RN, PhD, FAAN*
*Thelma Shobe Endowed Chair in Ethics and Spirituality in Nursing*
*University of California, School of Nursing, Department of Social and Behavioral Sciences*

# Contents

# PART TWO
## Career Planning Throughout Your Career

### Chapter Seven

# Taking Control of Your Nursing Career

## Second Edition

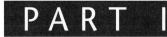

## PART I

# Career Planning and Development in Nursing

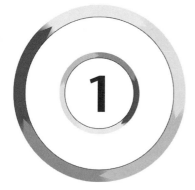

### Chapter One

# Taking Control of Your Nursing Career: The Future Is Now

Gail J. Donner, RN, PhD

**Gail J. Donner** is a partner in donnerwheeler, a consulting firm specializing in career planning and development, and Professor Emeritus in the Faculty of Nursing, University of Toronto. Gail's consulting and research interests are in career development, health policy, and nursing administration. She is active on boards and committees and has received numerous awards for her contributions to health care and the community.

## Author Reflections

*Mary and I decided to write this book because we believe that nurses want to take control of their careers and have the right to know how to do that and to be supported by colleagues as they do it. This book is one way Mary and I can fulfill our dream—a world in which each nurse is career resilient.*

*A career is an expression of how a person wants to be in the world.*

***Frederic Hudson***

Nursing has been marked by tremendous change in the last 50 years. It has been transformed from an occupation whose members struggled within a social context that devalued nurses' work as "women's work" to a profession composed of autonomous, well-educated, career-oriented knowledge workers. These changes have created new roles, new work settings, and new colleagues for nurses. Now we can work in a variety of settings—in institutions, in communities, and in independent businesses. We work alone, with other nurses, or in multidisciplinary teams in our roles as clinicians, educators, researchers, consultants, or managers. Moreover, nurses are presidents and chief executive officers of health care agencies, policy analysts, and politicians. All of these roles use the skills, knowledge, and spirit that nursing education and experience provide. These extraordinary changes have brought significant challenge along with terrific opportunity. As we have moved from thinking of and living with nursing as a job to considering nursing as a career, we have taken more charge of the profession and have begun to look at how to create futures for nurses as individuals and for the profession as a whole. This perceptual shift from viewing nursing as an episodic series of jobs to seeing it as a lifelong career has undoubtedly been the most significant change in nursing since Florence Nightingale professionalized nursing in the late 19th century.

The current health care environment poses a number of serious challenges for employers of nurses, and for other health care providers. The growing shortage of nurses, increasing reports of job dissatisfaction and low morale, and an aging nursing workforce are leading employers and policy-makers to identify nursing retention and recruitment as high priorities (Advisory Committee on Health Human Resources, 2002). What differentiates the current situation from past cycles of nursing shortages are the changes in the work environment that have resulted from organizational restructuring and increasing fiscal pressure on the system. Shortened hospital stays, sicker patients, heavier workloads, and increased use of unregulated workers have become common (Aiken et al., 2001; Fagin, 2001). These changes, along with a reduction of managers, educators, clinical nurse specialists, and other expert supports for nurses, have resulted in decreased job satisfaction, increased nurse illness and absenteeism, increased job stress, and demands for fundamental changes in work design. To support this urgent need to address working conditions, we now have mounting evidence about the impact of quality of work life on quality of patient care (Aiken, Sloane, & Sochalski, 1998; Baumann et al., 2001; Needleman et al., 2002).

As we enter the 21st century, a global shortage of nurses is becoming critical, and the major preoccupation of nurses' organizations, employers, governments, and other policy-makers is with strategies that enhance recruitment, retention, and the development of leadership capacity. At the same time, nurses are looking for workplaces that offer them stability with flexibility, policies that support continuing professional and educational development, and opportunities for career advancement. "What is apparent in all this work is the need not to repair nursing, but rather to renew and repair the work environments in which nurses practice. A growing body of evidence clearly supports the notion that making those changes does a great deal to recruit and retain the best nurses. In addition, it produces healthier and more satisfied patients and serves to attract and retain other health professionals who want to work in centres recognized for excellence as healthcare employers of choice" (Advisory Committee on Health Human Resources, 2002, p. 26).

Many factors influence a nurse's ability to thrive on the opportunities created and grow with change rather than merely react against it. Most nurses know they need to take control of their working lives and futures to make the most of change and to capitalize on new opportunities, but they often do not know where or how to begin. Career planning is a strategy that can offer nurses the means to respond to both short- and long-term changes in their profession and in the health care system. Career planning is "a continuous process of self-assessment and goal setting" (Kleinknecht & Hefferin, 1982, p. 31).

The process of planning and developing your career is an integral part of your ongoing professional development. Furthermore, the skills required to engage in career planning are the same skills nurses already use in their daily practice as part of problem solving and the nursing process. Just as you develop care plans with and for your patients, so too must you learn to design career plans for yourself and continuously monitor and evaluate your plans, revising each step of the process as necessary. The skills you rely on are the same, but the focus or target is different.

For more than 10 years the editors of this book have been consulting with nurses and employers of nurses in the area of career planning and development. Nurses have participated in our workshops and career coaching both onsite and online in Canada, the United States, Europe, and South Africa. The focus of our work has been to help nurses take charge of their careers and learn how to integrate career development into their ongoing professional and personal development. What we have learned is that nurses need and want help with this important part of their development; that they have dreams, goals, and ideas about their futures; and that they need a process to guide them in achieving those futures. The first edition of this book provided nurses with a model to use as a guide to their career development and with practical strategies for identifying and achieving success and satisfaction as they define it.

This new edition goes further in addressing the need to take control of your career, helping you understand why career planning is even more important now than it was in 1998, and equipping you with knowledge and skills to make career planning a part of your ongoing professional development. In this edition we provide you with an enhanced version of the Donner-Wheeler Career Planning and Development Model (Figure 1-1). We also provide a number of applications of the Model that reflect the diversity of career roles and opportunities that define nursing in the 21st century. As in the first edition, this book provides the tools to help you apply your understanding to your personal and professional environment. It is not meant to function as a quick fix or recipe book, but rather it offers an approach to living a rewarding and autonomous professional life. Although it is not specifically a job search book, many of the strategies presented will be invaluable in helping you find the job you want as a part of creating the career you deserve. It is written for every nurse—for those beginning a career in nursing and for those planning their retirement, for those wanting a change within nursing and for those contemplating a move away from nursing, for those who want to continue to work in organizations and for those who want to be independent practitioners, for those who love what they do and want to continue to do it, and for those who want to move in a new direction.

## THE STAGES OF A NURSING CAREER

Career planning can play a crucial role at every stage of one's career. In general, nurses' careers can be described as passing through five stages (Donner, 1992). Stage 1, *learning*, is the neophyte's introduction to nursing as a profession. It takes place within the basic educational program and is

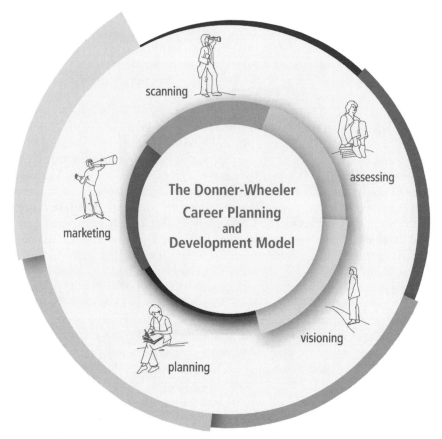

Figure **1-1.** Donner-Wheeler Career Planning and Development Model.

primarily concerned with learning "how to." Stage 2, the *entry phase*, begins when newly graduated nurses select their first workplace. It is that time of one's career when nurses explore their various employment options and begin to think about areas of practice that could be both appropriate and rewarding. In Stage 3, the *commitment phase*, nurses identify their likes and dislikes in terms of clinical areas, geography, work life, and other areas. At this point (usually anywhere from 2 to 5 years after graduation) nurses evaluate their career goals, seek mentors, consider continuing their education, and generally seek to find the right "fit" between themselves and their work settings. This is the time when nurses shift their focus from the job to a focus on career and long-term commitment. In Stage 4, the *consolidation phase*, nurses become comfortable with their chosen career path and with their relationship between the personal and the professional. This stage is notable for nurses' dedication to career, commitment to continuous learning, and focus on making a contribution to health care and to society. In this stage nurses begin to mentor others and to assume a leadership role in professional and community organizations. It is the longest stage in a nursing career, but it is certainly not a static one. In Stage 5, the *withdrawal stage*, nurses prepare for retirement and begin to think about what comes after nursing.

As you move through your career, your skills develop, your needs change, and your goals and plans evolve. Career planning is thus both important and useful at every stage of your career. It is a dynamic process that changes and adapts to changes in you and in the world in which you live and work. The career planning and development model that follows will provide you with a framework from which to grow and develop as a professional and to build your career in a comprehensive way.

## THE DONNER-WHEELER CAREER PLANNING AND DEVELOPMENT MODEL

Career development is a continuous process. Iterative rather than linear, it moves back and forth among phases rather than progressing in a lock-step linear fashion. It requires individuals to understand the environment in which they live and work, assess their own strengths and limitations and validate that assessment, articulate their personal career vision, develop a plan for the future that is realistic for them, and then market themselves to help achieve that plan. Simply put, it is a focused professional development strategy that helps nurses take greater responsibility for themselves and their careers and prepare for ever-changing health care systems and workplace environments. Career planning is something you engage in as part of your everyday professional activity. You can use it to help you stay happy and challenged with the work you are currently doing or to help you make a career change. The five phases of the model include the following:

**Phase One: Scanning Your Environment**
*What are the current realities/future trends?*

**Phase Two: Completing Your Self-Assessment and Reality Check**
*Who am I?*
*How do others see me?*

**Phase Three: Creating Your Career Vision**
*What do I really want to be doing?*

**Phase Four: Developing Your Strategic Career Plan**
*How can I achieve my career goals?*

**Phase Five: Marketing Yourself**
*How can I best market myself?*

### Scanning Your Environment

Scanning your environment can be described as taking stock of the world in which you live. It involves understanding the current realities in the health care system and the work environment, as well as understanding the future trends at the global, national, and local levels both within and outside of health care and the nursing profession. Through the scanning process you become better informed, learn to see the world through differing perspectives, and are able to identify current and future career opportunities. Scanning is a continuous activity that, together with self-assessment, forms the foundation of the career planning process. We observe, learn about, and assess the world around us through reading, talking with others, continuing our education, and exposing ourselves to information and ideas—not only from and about nursing and health care but also from other disciplines and ideologies. With this solid understanding of our environment, we go on to complete a self-assessment.

## Completing Your Self-Assessment and Reality Check

If an environmental scan is about looking outside into the world, then a self-assessment is about looking inside yourself. Just as you would not consider developing a patient care plan without a thorough patient assessment, so it is with career planning. A thorough self-assessment is the key to exploring new and previously unconsidered opportunities. It enables you to identify your values, experiences, knowledge, strengths, and limitations and to marry those with your environmental scan to create your career vision and to identify the direction to take as you plan your future. Just as we seek validation in our patient assessments, so too should we complete a reality check of our self-assessment. A reality check is simply about seeking feedback regarding our strengths and limitations—about expanding our view of ourselves through reflecting on others' perspectives.

## Creating Your Career Vision

Once you have determined a realistic and comprehensive picture of your own values, beliefs, and skills and have assessed these in the context of the real world scan you have completed, you are ready to think about your career possibilities. What is it that you really want for yourself? Where do you see yourself going? Do you like what you are currently doing, believe it is a good fit with your personal life, and want to grow and develop within that role? Or have you learned that you enjoy change and variety and that it may be time to move on to other challenges? Because your vision of your potential future is grounded in your scan and self-assessment, it is focused on what is possible and realistic for you, both short-term and long-term. Your career vision is the link between who you are and what you can become.

## Developing Your Strategic Career Plan

A strategic career plan is a blueprint for action. According to Barker (1992), vision without action is only a dream; action without vision only passes the time; but vision with action can change the world. Now you are ready to specify the activities, timelines, and resources you need to help you achieve your goals and career vision. This is the part of the process where you start to put on paper the specific strategies you will use to take charge of your future. Of course, this is also where the spiral or iterative nature of the process is reinforced. For example, you may have planned to do some diabetic teaching with your patient at a specific time in the morning, but if you enter the room or the home and see a very anxious and distraught patient with a nearly hysterical family at the bedside, you undoubtedly reassess your plan and adapt it to the current environment. So it is with career planning. We should be constantly scanning our environment, assessing ourselves, and re-evaluating our goals and plans for reaching them.

### Marketing Yourself

Just as you help your patients articulate their needs to achieve their health goals, so must you learn to speak for yourself so that you can successfully implement your career plans. Regardless of whether you have chosen the traditional nursing role as an employee or have decided to embark on self-employment, you will need to acquire marketing skills.

Marketing involves the ability to package your professional and personal qualities, attributes, and expertise so that you can effectively communicate— to your employer or client—what you have to offer and why you are the best person for the service that needs to be delivered.

As a nurse, marketing yourself is facilitated by establishing a network, acquiring a mentor, and developing your written and verbal communication skills. Thus self-marketing entails scanning the environment and "knowing your business." Having the ability to articulate who you are, what you want, and what you can do represents only half the equation. The other half is the ability to persuade others that what you can offer meets the demands and challenges of the ever-changing environment.

## HOW TO USE THIS BOOK

This book is a guide that you should each use in the way that best suits your learning style. Career planning is a serious process that takes time and perseverance. We have organized this second edition to enable you to learn as much as you can about the career planning process and our Model and then to help you apply the Model to your particular interests and life/career stage. Part One provides you with a comprehensive overview of the five phases of the Model along with examples to help you understand and apply each phase. Linda McGillis Hall begins this section with a discussion of scanning and a scan of the current environment to help you understand the world of health and health care and to provide you with a guide or template for doing your own scanning. Gail Donner asks the questions you need to consider to assess who you are and what you have to offer. Mary Wheeler then shows you how to match your environmental scan with your self-assessment to create your personal career vision. Armed with that vision, you are now able, with

Claire Mallette's help, to determine your career goals and design your own strategic career plan to achieve those goals. Finally, Sue Bookey-Bassett provides you with insight and strategies on using marketing to achieve your plan.

After completing Part One, you should have a pretty clear idea about where you want to go and how you think you might get there.

Part Two helps you focus on the career continuum. You can either read the rest of the book in a continuous way or, if you prefer, you can go directly to specific chapters or sections to get help with your particular learning and career needs. Part Two begins with a chapter by Janice Waddell that focuses on helping students learn how to adapt the career planning process to their particular needs. To supplement this book, *Building Your Nursing Career* (2004) provides a comprehensive guide specifically for nursing students. It helps students learn to use their student clinical experiences along with their non-nursing experiences and expertise to help achieve their career goals. Mary Wheeler's chapter helps the mid-career nurse understand what is happening at this life and career stage and provides strategies and tools to assist mid-career nurses in identifying and reclaiming what they really want. For those of you who are approaching retirement and who want to think about that phase of your life and career in a proactive way, Margot Young provides the help you need to create your own retirement agenda. One of the benefits that the ever-changing health care environment has yielded is the opportunity for nurses to pursue independent practice. Michelle Cooper, an entrepreneur, applies the Model to entrepreneurial and intrapreneurial practice. The strategies she provides will help you as you plan to move to the world of independent practice or to stay inside organizations where intrapreneurship is promoted and valued.

Part Three is devoted to the future in career planning and development and to the need for it to be embedded and integrated into organizational cultures, policies, and processes. Since the first edition of this book, we have seen career planning and development emerge as a valuable strategy for creating quality workplace and practice environments and for recruiting and retaining nurses. We close the book with a recipe for the creation of a career development culture as part of creating the desired future for nurses and nursing.

## TAKING CONTROL

Attending to your professional development is a time-intensive process that requires both reflection and planning. The career planning process presented in this book gives you a way to relate your ideas and vision to the practical realities of your life and achieve useful and realizable outcomes. It represents an approach that allows you to get the most out of yourself and your career while you give the most to your clients. The career planning process is really about the development of a life skill—one that you can apply not only in your workplace but also in your personal life. The process described in this book is not magical, nor is it relevant only for nurses. Although it can be used as a personal guide, it can also be shared with family and friends. A career needs attention and nurturing. This book is intended to provide you with the skills you need to care for yourself and your career. Your future is in your hands!

## REFERENCES

Advisory Committee on Health Human Resources (October 2002). *Our health, our future: Creating quality workplaces for Canadian nurses.* Ottawa, Ontario, Canada: Author. Updated November 23, 2002. http://www.hc-sc.gc.ca/English/for_you/nursing/cnac_report/index.html

Aiken, L.H., Sloane, D.M., & Sochalski, J. (1998). Hospital organization and outcomes. *Quality in Health Care, 7*(4), 222-226.

Aiken, L., et al. (2001). Nurses' reports on hospital care in five countries. *Health Affairs, 20*(3), 43-53.

Barker, J. (1992). *Paradigms: The business of discovering the future.* New York: Harper Collins.

Baumann, A., et al. (2001). *Commitment and care: The benefits of a healthy workplace for nurses, their patients and the system.* Report submitted to the Canadian Health Services Research Foundation, Ottawa, Ontario, Canada. Updated November 11, 2002. http://www.chsrf.ca/docs/finalrpts/psomcare_e.pdf

Donner, G.J. (1992). Career development and mobility issues. In A. Baumgart, & J. Larsen (Eds.), *Canadian nursing faces the future* (2nd ed., pp. 345-363). St. Louis: Mosby.

Fagin, C.M. (2001). When care becomes a burden: Diminishing access to adequate nursing. *Milbank Memorial Fund.* Retrieved December 12, 2002. http://www.milbank.org/010216fagin.html

Kleinknecht, M.K., & Hefferin, E.A. (1982). Assisting nurses toward professional growth: A career development model. *Journal of Nursing Administration, 12*(5), 30-36.

Needleman, J., et al. (2002). Nurse-staffing levels and the quality of care in hospitals. *The New England Journal of Medicine, 346*(22), 1715-1722.

Waddell, J., Donner, G.J., & Wheeler, M.M. (2004). *Building your nursing career.* Toronto, Ontario, Canada: Elsevier.

## FURTHER READING

Moses, B. (2000). *The good news about careers: how you'll be working in the next decade.* San Francisco: Jossey-Bass.

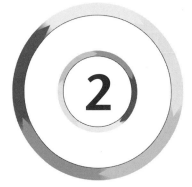

# Beginning the Process: Scanning Your Environment

Linda McGillis Hall, RN, MSc, PhD

**Linda McGillis Hall** is an Assistant Professor at the Faculty of Nursing, University of Toronto. She is also a New Investigator with the Canadian Institutes of Health Research and a Co-Investigator with the Nursing Effectiveness, Utilization, and Outcomes Research Unit—a joint project between the University of Toronto and McMaster University. Linda's publications are primarily in the area of nursing administration and staff mix. She is also an Associate with donnerwheeler.

## Author Reflections

*As a nurse researcher, scanning helps me understand the context of the nursing work environment. It helps me keep my career situated in the present and focused on the future.*

*It was the best of times; it was the worst of times.*

**Charles Dickens**

When asked to think about the word *environment*, you should conjure up not only a close-up picture of the setting in which health care is practiced, but also a wide-angle shot of the broader area surrounding you—that is, the external conditions within which you live. Just as you would not consider providing care to clients without knowing something about their family and socioeconomic circumstances and their health status, so too you must think about the broader context of your external environment before you can understand how current trends and future developments in health care could affect your career. Scanning the environment and completing a self-assessment form the foundation of the career planning process. Scanning provides you with the information you need to understand your current world and to identify possible opportunities and options for developing your career in the future. You must have a solid understanding of the environment before you can decide how to use your skills and experience in a way that is most beneficial for you and for society.

In this chapter you will learn about the scanning process—what it is, why it is important, and how to do it. This chapter then provides you with a scan of some key issues in the current health care environment and concludes with some help so that you can begin your own scanning activity.

## THE WHAT, WHY, AND HOW OF SCANNING

Scanning is the easiest and most productive way to place yourself as an observer, rather than a player, in the world in which you live. It permits you to see beyond your immediate circumstances to grasp what is possible, to think about new things in new ways, and to open yourself to opportunities without any censoring of ideas. Scanning provides you with the information you need to understand your own reality and to identify possible short-term and long-term opportunities for your career. A comprehensive knowledge of the environment is the foundation you need to be able to determine how to use your skills and experience to benefit both you and society.

If we are to understand what is happening now and what may be happening in the future, each of us must scan continuously and in a variety of ways throughout our careers. Sources of information include professional and popular journals, observation, print, other forms of new media, friends and colleagues, and everyday experiences. The Internet is a new and highly valuable instrument to help you scan. It allows you to read the news; survey the various professional organizations; access policy papers, journals, and other resources; and communicate with colleagues around the world. Think of all the means you use to understand the context in which you deliver care to clients, and then apply those means to learning about your own environment.

Reading, talking, and listening—skills that nurses have as part of their repertoire of behaviours—are the means we use to make sense of all of the information we collect. Consider your scan as a work in progress and as something you continuously update and revise to reflect the changing environment. Scanning is not a task to be completed at some regular or not-so-regular time; rather it is an integral part of everyday professional and personal life.

## A BEGINNING SCAN OF TODAY'S HEALTH CARE ENVIRONMENT

Because the health care environment is constantly changing, what follows is a sample of a scan of today's environment done at a particular point in time. This scan is provided as an example of what a scan looks like and is intended to help you get started. Of course, when you do your own scan you should consider not only the health care environment but also the social, political, and economic environments. Often these environments not only affect health care but also influence the number and range of available career opportunities.

Think of your scan as written in pencil, not in ink, and as something you continuously revise to reflect the changing environment. If you are prepared in that way, you should be able to identify the global, national, and local trends and issues at any given time. You can then use your scan to help you position yourself and your career for your future.

## Key Issues in Health Care

The world seems a smaller place today as access to information about our world is readily at hand. Global health concerns and trends are often also national and sometimes even local issues. For example, infectious diseases (including AIDS), resource allocation, the gap between rich and poor, the changing health care system, and the shortage of nurses are predominant health and social issues in almost every country. In this scan, we focus on a few key issues with significant implications for nursing and for nurses.

### The Shortage of Nurses

As we approached the 21st century, the market for nursing services was uncertain, and many nurses in all walks of nursing life had experienced layoffs or enforced early retirement—often an entirely new experience for them. Predictably, the tremendous cuts in nursing positions marked the beginning of serious nursing workforce issues. In Canada, for example, the number of registered nurses employed in nursing declined annually by 2.5% from 1994 to 1999 (Canadian Institute for Health Information, 2000).

Although nursing shortages have been experienced in the past, a number of new phenomena occurring simultaneously may have a greater influence on the shortages of nurses today. These phenomena include declining enrollments in nursing, poor retention of nurses in their workplaces, and early retirement (Berliner & Ginzberg, 2002). In the United States, the passage of the Nurse Reinvestment Act was intended to support individuals entering nursing through scholarships and loans. The Act, which provides funding opportunities for nurses and may aid in reducing the shortage, is one of the new strategies being used to facilitate recruitment to nursing. In Canada, vigorous media campaigns extolling the benefits of a nursing career have been adopted, and the profession has been positioned as influential in determining the future of health care.

In the United States, the magnet hospital movement has drawn considerable attention as a strategy to help us understand what characterizes a quality work environment for nurses (Trossman, 2002). Creative strategies to improve recruitment and retention have become the focus of considerable attention by policy-makers, employers, and researchers (Advisory Committee on Health Human Resources, 2002; Newman & Maylor, 2002; Shiels & Ward, 2001).

Although the nursing shortage provides a big challenge for employers and educators, it also creates opportunity for nurses. When demand for our services is high, we can choose the employment that best fits our values and needs. For example, we can look at alternative career choices (e.g., entrepreneurship or a role in complementary therapies) or consider leadership opportunities that might not have been there in the past.

### The Rise of Consumer-Driven Models

Another significant shift in health care in many countries is the move from provider-driven models of health care delivery to consumer-driven models. As in the business environment, customer satisfaction became a key issue, and consumers were emerging as the dominant force in the health care provider–consumer relationship. They have become more educated about the health care choices and alternatives available to them and are demanding a health care system that is configured to their needs. Evidence of consumer involvement in health care includes the development of patients' rights statements, legislation relating to consumer advocacy, and a trend toward increasing the role and numbers of consumers as trustees on boards of health care agencies. Mechanisms to elicit and assess patient satisfaction became common in health care organizations, and patient representative roles emerged in an effort to help identify and manage patient concerns regarding health care practices.

The rise of consumer-driven models is a wonderful complement to the nursing role and provides a variety of career opportunities, such as becoming more involved in advocacy, partnering with patients to achieve health care reform, and becoming more involved in policy work.

### Influences of Technology

The tremendous technological advances in health care that have been occurring simultaneously have had a marked effect on health care and have added to consumer expectations of the health care system. For example, many illnesses are being treated today that could not even be diagnosed in the past. Great progress has been made in the areas of organ transplantation and non-invasive and microscopic surgery. These technological advances are expensive and have created a pyramid effect that has had a dramatic impact on overall health care costs. They have also created a paradox for health care officials who must constantly weigh the interests of the consumer against the costs of providing the care. Nursing roles have evolved as nurses have developed the technical expertise needed to manage patients—both in hospitals and in the community—after undergoing these complex procedures and treatments.

In addition, computerization has had significant effects on health care and on nursing practice. It will continue to pose a challenge for nurses as we learn to understand both the computer's potential to influence our practice and its larger role in health care delivery. This challenge represents a great opportunity for nurses who see the computer as a friend; they can act as valuable resources to nurses who are uncomfortable with the prospect of increasing computerization.

### Health Care in the Community

In the developed world, community health has been slow to emerge because the focus of health care has been primarily institutional or hospital-based. Traditionally, community health settings emphasize preventive medicine and health promotion rather than the episodic, curative approaches to health care that are common in hospital settings. Over the past few years, however, a great deal of interest has been directed toward enhancing community health.

As hospitals have begun to look at alternatives to cut the costs of patient care, the most prevalent response has been shortened lengths of stay. The consequence of this trend is a corresponding increase in the need for patient care within the community. However, it has been difficult to adapt traditional community nursing practice patterns to accommodate these changes, especially without the ability to increase nursing staff volumes. Once again, expert hospital nurses have a tremendous opportunity to develop their careers by devising responses to these challenges to meet the needs of both the new community and the hospital sector. In addition, the role of the primary care nurse practitioner provides nurses the opportunity to expand their practice while working with physicians in a collaborative role in the community. Recent data indicate that, although the majority of nurses in Canada continue to work in hospitals, the number employed in community health is gradually increasing (Canadian Institutes of Health Information, 2001). In the United States, the increasing role of nurse practitioners has also expanded the opportunity for nurses to provide service to clients in a wide range of settings outside hospitals. In other countries, the provision of nursing and health services to large populations has been the almost exclusive territory of nurses.

### Changes in the Workplace

The structural reforms in health care being implemented throughout the world have been accompanied by many changes in the workplace or at the local level. Structural changes resulting from mergers, regionalization, restructuring, and managed care have led to changes both in the roles of management and staff in health care organizations and in the relationships between employers and employees.

*The Changing Employer-Employee Relationship.* The changes in employer-employee relationships, which are pervasive at the workplace level, is perhaps also the biggest system-wide change that has influenced nursing and health care and is part of the general global reorganization of work. Some of the reasons for these changes are the high costs associated with the allocation of human resources, the introduction of technology, and evolving social values. The old relationship was long-term and full-time. Reward for performance was a promotion; loyalty guaranteed a lifetime career, and experience and education were key factors in upward mobility.

Nurses in the old relationship entered an organization confident that they would have a position for life if they remained loyal and did their work satisfactorily. Indeed, organizations had a variety of lower stress and less physical roles (e.g., procedure manual coordinator or staffing coordinator) that were available to older, loyal nurse employees. These positions no longer exist. In the new relationships, roles and positions are situational, systems are temporary, and positions are often short-term, contract, or part-time. Reward for performance is acknowledgement of contribution, loyalty means responsibility and good work, and rapidly evolving skills are needed. Nurses are employed for the work that needs doing and have little guarantee of longevity in the organization.

Although stressful and frightening for nurses who have been in health care for a number of years, these changes are more popular among younger Generation-X'ers (26- to 35-year-olds), who see them as providing room for autonomy and opportunity. It is even more likely that these changes will not be enough for the Generation-Y'ers (16- to 25-year-olds) who grew up in the information age with access to the world at their fingertips through television, the Internet, and instant communication. Although there may have been a sense of security in the old dependent relationship, there was also lack of freedom to determine one's own future. The new relationship can provide opportunities to enhance control over your future.

Nurses are typical of other "new" employees in this changed environment. They are looking for workplaces that offer stability with flexibility, policies that support continuing professional and educational development, and opportunities for career advancement. As short-sighted solutions fail to meet their needs, difficulties retaining and recruiting into both the profession and the workplace remain. Finding long-term, viable solutions to this dilemma is becoming increasingly vital as mounting evident connects issues of workload, staffing, and job satisfaction with quality patient care. For the first time, a growing number of reliable studies point to a definitive relationship between quality of work life and quality of care. Because addressing workforce issues is not an option anymore, work design, professional development, and opportunities for career advancement are beginning to receive the attention they deserve. Chapter 11 provides more information about current workplace environments and how we might improve those environments for nurses.

*The Changing Role of Nurse Executives.* Business processes have been used to redesign and flatten the structure of health care organizations. Departments have been reconfigured into patient service areas that are organized by programs or grouped by patient diagnosis. To support this orientation toward patients, existing departments are redistributed within these programs. One of the most significant shifts has been in nursing, where entire nursing departments have been abolished and nursing has been dispersed into individual patient service groupings. In many cases the profession of nursing has been relabelled as a service occupation within the organizational structure. Once the nursing service has been redistributed and the nursing department dissolved, there is no longer a role for a department head of nursing. In a recent study of 29 teaching hospitals across nine census regions of the United States, 97% of the sites reported that the chief nurse executive position had been transformed from a nursing executive to a patient care executive (Sovie & Jawad, 2001). In most reconfigured institutions, it was still thought necessary to have some role for a nursing leader in the organizational chart, because nurses remain the largest provider group for patient care in hospitals. What often results is the position of chief of nursing practice, which entails little if any fiscal power or authority. Some see this dissolution of nursing departments as a serious threat to the status and influence of nursing in the hospital and as the first step in the systematic weakening of nursing's role of patient care management in hospitals.

*The Changing Role of Unit Managers.* The concerted effort to apply business principles to health care is also reflected in the changes that have occurred in the role requirements for the manager of these reconfigured patient care units. The increased span of control, the increasing focus on budget, and the availability of less time to provide leadership and guidance to staff are key features of the unit manager position today. Along with this change has come the demand for more education. Both employers and prospective managers want more preparation, and graduate education in nursing and/or business administration is quickly becoming a minimum requirement for management at the unit level.

*The Effect of Changes in the Workplace on the Role and Future of the Nurse.* Health care reforms and the resulting changes to the health care system and the workplace provide a unique set of challenges and potential opportunities for the registered nurse. Despite the restructuring and redesign initiatives that have taken place, the role of the registered nurse in providing patient care has remained constant. Although some structural changes within health care appear to devolve the role of nurses in the health care system, these may in effect lead to a more substantive recognition of the importance of the registered nurse's role in patient care delivery. As consumers become more educated and involved in patient care within this reformed system, they are demanding more in-depth explanations of their care processes and of outcomes they can expect to achieve. Answers to these questions will require knowledge. Drucker (1980) suggested that the workforce is composed of two segments of workers: knowledge workers and service workers. Knowledge workers are those with fairly advanced educations who perform highly specialized tasks and enjoy unlimited mobility compared to service workers. The registered nurse is fast becoming the knowledge worker in this reformed health care system.

In the new organizational structures, care providers also have limited direction, guidance, or supervision from their managers. Support roles that existed in former care delivery models have been deleted. Staff responsible for patient care will be required to be independent, autonomous thinkers who are capable of making decisions on their own, have experience doing so, and have been educated to do so as part of their professional practice.

One of the challenges for registered nurses is coping with the fragmented employment pattern that exists in the current economy. Considering the increased level of patient involvement in the health care system, however, patients may soon respond to the lack of continuity and inconsistency in treatment and care planning that occurs when a full-time labour force is not utilized. From patients' perspectives, the use of temporary or part-time workers may prove more costly than cost efficient.

Patients also value and recognize registered nurses for their knowledge. It does not really matter whether nursing is nestled within its own division, programs, or in patient groupings within an organizational structure. Registered nurses are the only care providers who possess the knowledge and skill to support the new structures that have been created in response to these system reforms. In a recent Gallup poll in the United States, nursing was rated by almost 8 in 10 Americans as the profession with the highest standards of honesty and ethics.

## NOW IT IS YOUR TURN

Having seen an example of a scan, it is now time to try to do one yourself. Figure 2-1 provides you with a template for scanning your own environment. It begins by asking you to consider what you see globally, then nationally and, finally, locally. Although there is considerable overlap between these trends, it is helpful to try to think about the issues in this way. Once you have done your scan, consider which of those issues and trends are specifically meaningful for you in your own personal and professional environments. The trends and issues you identify in your scan will serve as a basis for you to make informed decisions about potential career opportunities. Remember that you will need to review and revise your scan on a regular basis.

## CONCLUSION

Scanning teaches us that although these are somewhat unsettled times, the career opportunities for nurses to demonstrate leadership in innovative approaches to quality care are limitless. The trends and issues you identify in your scan will serve as a basis for you to make informed decisions about career options and then to plan strategically to implement them. Before you begin to put your plan into place, you need to turn your sights inward and do a thorough self-assessment. This is the subject of Chapter 3.

| Global Trends and Issues | | |
|---|---|---|
| Society | Health Care | Nursing |
| | | |

| National Trends and Issues | | |
|---|---|---|
| Society | Health Care | Nursing |
| | | |

| Local Trends and Issues | | |
|---|---|---|
| Society | Health Care | Nursing |
| | | |

Figure **2-1.** Scanning your environment.

# REFERENCES

Advisory Committee on Health Human Resources (October 2002). *Our health, our future: Creating quality workplaces for Canadian nurses.* Ottawa, Ontario, Canada: Author. Updated November 23, 2002. http://www.hc-sc.gc.ca/English/for_you/nursing/cnac_report/index.html

Berliner, H.S., & Ginzberg, E. (2002). Why this hospital nursing shortage in different. *Journal of the American Medical Association, 288*(21), 2742-2744.

Canadian Institute of Health Information. (2000). *Supply and distribution of registered nurses in Canada, 1999.* Ottawa, Ontario, Canada: Author.

Canadian Institute of Health Information. (2001). *Canada's health care providers.* Ottawa, Ontario, Canada: Author.

Drucker, P. (1980). *Managing in turbulent times.* New York: Harper & Row.

Newman, K., & Maylor, U. (2002). The NHS plan: Nurse satisfaction, commitment and retention strategies. *Health Services Management Research, 15*(20), 93-105.

Shiels, M.A., & Ward, M. (2001). Improving nurse retention in the National Health Service in England: The impact of job satisfaction on intentions to quit. *Journal of Health Economics, 20*(5), 677-701.

Sovie, M.D., & Jawad, A.F. (2001). Hospital restructuring and its impact on outcomes. *Journal of Nursing Administration, 31*(12), 588-600.

Trossman, S. (2002). Nursing magnets: Attracting talent and making it stick. Magnet hospitals stem the nursing shortage with better recruitment and retention. *American Journal of Nursing, 1022,* 87-89.

# FURTHER READING

Hammer, M., & Champy, J. (1993). *Reengineering the corporation.* New York: Harper Collins.

McGillis Hall, L. (1997). Staff mix models: Complementary or substitution roles for nurses. *Nursing Administration Quarterly, 21*(2), 31-39.

Shortell, S.M., et al. (1996). *Remaking health care in America: Building organized delivery systems.* San Francisco: Jossey-Bass.

World Health Organization. (2001). *Public service reforms and their impact on health sector personnel.* Geneva, Switzerland: World Health Organization, International Labour Office.

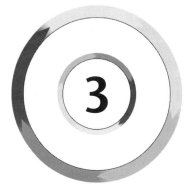

# Completing Your Self-Assessment and Reality Check

Gail J. Donner, RN, PhD

Gail J. Donner, RN, PhD

---

**▌Author Reflections**

*It's amazing how much taking time to think about what's important to me has been critical in helping me decide what path to take. If I had to identify one thing that has made my career so exciting and so rewarding, it has been my continuous exploration of who I am and what is important to me.*

*Real value...can only be given by people who know their own value. How can any of us know our true value if we never take inventory?*

**John Scherer**

Now that you have scanned the environment, learned what surrounds you, and understand what that told you about the present, the future, and potential career opportunities, it is time to turn the focus on yourself. As you begin your self-assessment, you will first identify all the attributes that make you who you are and what you have to offer to the environment. Completing your self-assessment allows you to give honest and accurate answers to the two questions: "Who am I?" and "How am I seen?" When put together with the results of your environmental scan, your replies will enable you to complete the last three phases of the career planning and development process: creating your career vision, developing your strategic career plan, and marketing yourself. Scanning your environment and completing your self-assessment and reality check are pivotal to being able to ask yourself that final question: "What, then, shall I plan to do?"

This chapter addresses the process of self-assessment, why it is important, and how to accomplish it. As with scanning, self-assessment should not be a one-time activity, but rather a continuous part of your personal and professional development. The sooner you begin a systematic process of self-assessment—whether you are in your first year of nursing, an experienced practitioner, or someone contemplating retirement—the more attuned and meaningful will be the match between you and the work you do.

## WHY DO A SELF-ASSESSMENT?

"If life is to have meaning the extent to which you know yourself is the most important work you will ever do. And because life is a process of emergence and becoming, it is a journey, not a destination" (Crow, 2000, p. 15). Whether the job market is tight or whether jobs are plentiful, individuals must be able to recognize their skills and take the initiative to market these skills to prospective employers. Before they hire you, employers want to examine—in more depth than ever before—who you are and what you can do for them. You need to be able to articulate your accomplishments clearly and persuasively so they reveal your values, skills, and interests. That is what completing a self-assessment does; it involves giving yourself the time and permission to concentrate and look inward, take stock, and develop a personal and professional profile. Self-assessment requires considerable reflection, the ability to ask yourself some hard questions, and the determination to validate your responses with others. And it must become an ongoing process in your continuous professional and personal learning and development.

Over the years you have likely gathered some impressions about what you like or dislike doing and have acquired some sense of your abilities and limitations. You may also have developed in many ways outside your professional arena. After these experiences, who you are now may be very different from who you were when you chose nursing as a career. However, without a deliberate and systematic self-assessment, you can at best have only a fuzzy picture of your current self. How, then, can you know what you want and are best able to do now, let alone how to take control to direct your future? If you neglect this phase in the career planning and development process, you will be driven only by the needs of the market or the opinions of others. The result is often dissatisfaction with the job chosen or poor performance because your values, knowledge, skills, and interests do not match the job requirements.

> Without completing a thorough self-assessment, Carlotta, a staff nurse, would not have an accurate way to determine whether her 8 years of experience in the Neonatal Intensive Care Unit actually suited her to become the nurse manager in that unit. She knew that even though she did an excellent job at the bedside, it did not necessarily follow that she had the values, knowledge, skills, and interests required to perform successfully in a management position.

Although completing a self-assessment takes time, the result is a better awareness of you and your strengths and limitations. The process will help you learn about which facets of yourself have remained unexpressed or untapped and how to develop them. Moreover, you will begin to understand how you may be limited by learned perceptions, familiar but unsatisfying roles, or others' expectations. You will then be better able to capitalize on your strengths and life experiences.

Make sure that your self-assessment is comprehensive. Think about who you are from a number of perspectives. How would you describe your personality, your attitude, how you work with others, and your comfort with communication? Self-assessment is as much about your personal qualities and special interests as it is about your professional knowledge and clinical skills. Employers are increasingly interested in a broad range of skills. Therefore the more comprehensive you can be about who you are—the person and the professional—the better able you will be to market yourself when you need to do so.

Once you have completed your self-assessment, you will be able to promote what you have to offer and will understand where you need to improve or add to your knowledge and skills. With an accurate picture of yourself to add to your environmental scan, you will be able to investigate the full spectrum of available opportunities and decide which options are the right ones for you. Your confidence and self-esteem will soar.

## COMPLETING YOUR SELF-ASSESSMENT

### Who Am I?

Work is just one part of our lives, but regrettably many people describe who they are only in relation to the work they do. Answering this question involves much more than stating your job title or describing what you do. Even though we spend a considerable amount of time at a job, we cannot ignore the other components that complete our lives, including our health, financial resources, friends, family, and community. As you move through your self-assessment, you need to keep the whole you in mind. Think, for instance, about all the adjectives you could use to detail what makes you unique. Although we are all unique and special, the challenge lies in being able to articulate that uniqueness.

For many nurses, these activities are not easy. How often have you overheard colleagues respond with, "Oh, I'm just a nurse," when asked to tell about themselves? But no one is "just" anything. We are complex human beings, the sum of our past and current experiences, whose selves are composed of mind, body, emotions, and spirit. Maslow (1970) coined the term *self-actualization*, which is the ability to realize one's potential capacities by becoming involved in pursuits that engage all four aspects of self in a balanced way that leads to a meaningful life.

Who we are includes our beliefs and values, our knowledge, our skills, and our interests. Beliefs are the way in which we view ourselves and the world around us. Values are a set of beliefs that drive our decisions, actions, behaviours, and relations. They are the ideals that guide and give meaning to our lives and work. Recognizing your knowledge and skills and the degree to which you possess them are crucial outcomes of the self-assessment process. Knowledge is gained through formal and informal education and through work and life experiences. It is the foundation from which your nursing practice develops. Skills are the abilities and behaviours we use to produce results, and interests are the activities in which we like to spend most of our time and from which we gain pleasure.

Completing a self-assessment to discover who you are is like looking at a tapestry—rich in the colours and designs that reflect all of you. It will show you where you have been and where you are now, both personally and professionally. Just as your self continues to unfold and grow in a lifelong process, so too must your self-assessment be a continuous part of your development activities throughout your career as new experiences are woven into the ever-growing tapestry.

## BEGINNING THE PROCESS

As you proceed with your self-assessment, you will begin to recognize some common themes and patterns that have shaped who you are and what you do. You will also be able to identify clearly what you value, as well as your interests, special talents, and abilities. You can then begin to spot any lack of congruence between them and your current activities and perhaps start to get a picture of where you may like to be in the future.

Figure 3-1 provides some preliminary questions that can help you understand who you are and what is important to you. These questions should not limit you but should act as a catalyst to start your reflections. Your answers will give you the words to describe your unique self, what you like to do, and what you have to offer. This is a good time to begin a journal—a record of your progress as you grow and a means to keep track of thoughts and ideas you have along your journey (James-Neill, 1982). Recording your responses in a journal provides you with tangible evidence of who you are. As you start to document your answers, you can begin to write your own story: where you have been, where you are now, and what you have learned about yourself along the way. Your story should include all the important personal and professional events in your life and how they relate to one another. As you write your story, envision that you are writing your autobiography. What would you call it? Could you locate the chapter you are in now, and what title would you give it? As you move forward in the career planning and development process, keep your journal handy to consult and to add or delete information as needed.

### Assessing Your Values

Values are those principles we prize, cherish, or esteem—those beliefs we hold as extremely important. Values direct our decisions and influence our lives. Psychologists suggest that ultimate satisfaction comes from living and working in concert with our values. As you begin to identify your values, consider which ones are present in your current job or role and which ones are not. Three questions will help you get started: (1) What is important to me in my job and in my personal life?, (2) Where are my priorities—self, family, community, or other?, and (3) Who or what are the significant things that I

---

## WHO AM I?

### Values
- What is important to me in my job and in my personal life?
- Who or what are the significant people or things I need to consider at this time?
- Where are my priorities: self, family, community, other?

### Knowledge
- What is my formal education? What specialty or other certification do I hold?
- What is my area of expertise?
- How has that expertise been developed through my work experience?
- Describe your expertise in one sentence: I am knowledgeable about _____.
- What knowledge requires further development?

### Skills
List your skills, being as comprehensive and specific as you can. Categories may include clinical skills, interpersonal skills, teaching skills, communication skills, and other skills.
- What are my strengths? My limitations?
- What skills require further development?

### Interests
- What have I liked about my job(s)/role(s)?
- What haven't I liked?
- What energizes or motivates me?
- What do I like to do outside of the workplace?
- In what type of environment do I perform my best?

### Accomplishments
- What are my three most significant accomplishments at work over the past 2 to 3 years?
- What are my three most significant accomplishments outside of work?
- List three times you believe you have made a difference.

---

Figure **3-1.** Completing your self-assessment.

need to consider at this time in my life? For example, if you are at a stage in your personal life where you are considering starting a family, you should think about how this decision will affect your career. If your workplace is changing the role of manager so that it no longer includes a clinical component, you need to consider whether that is still congruent with what you believe the role of manager should be. Finally, if the opportunity to learn is important to you, a workplace that offers a means of continuing your education, either formally or informally, will be of greater value to you.

## Assessing Your Knowledge

Our knowledge develops through the combination of formal learning and experience. As you consider the knowledge you have acquired, you will benefit by reviewing your past education (including the degrees, diplomas, and specialty certificates you have acquired) and the workshops and seminars you have attended. What is your area of expertise? How has that expertise been developed through your work experience? Complete the sentence, "I am knowledgeable about_____," or "I have expertise in_____."

## Assessing Your Skills

Skills are developed or acquired abilities. There are three general categories of skills: (1) technical or job content or "hard skills," such as those involved with providing total nursing care to neonates; (2) managerial skills, which concern communication, coordination, or support; and (3) personal traits, such as adaptability, energy, or logical reasoning. Managerial skills and personal traits would be considered "soft skills" and often are highly transferable.

In this component of the self-assessment process, you should evaluate both your hard and soft skills and understand what you have to offer a potential employer. Take some time to reflect on your entire career, and consider the most significant highlights or milestones along the way. Consider not only the professional work you have done, but also the skills you have developed outside of your work as a nurse, perhaps as a community volunteer or as a parent. Identifying the skills you have acquired will enable you to clarify what you have to offer and to determine which skills can be transferred to other settings. Skills such as case management, documentation, problem solving, and crisis management are generic skills that can easily be transferred to a variety of roles and organizations, both within and outside of health care. Which of your skills require further development? Skill gaps or limitations are just as important to acknowledge as your strengths. If you do not recognize these limitations and act to address them, you may assume roles for which you are ill suited and thereby inhibit your ability to succeed.

## Assessing Your Interests

Interests provide another measure of "fit" between what a job provides and what we would ideally like to be doing. They can be grouped into four categories: (1) people—helping, serving, caring for, or selling things to people; (2) data—working with facts, records, or files; (3) things—working with machines, tools, or living things; and (4) ideas—creating insights, theories, or new ways of saying or doing something. Think about the work you have done and the life you have lived. What energizes or motivates you? What do you enjoy in your current work? What haven't you liked? In what type of environment do you perform at your best? What type of people do you like to have around you? What habits and styles of learning appeal to you? For instance, if working with technology and equipment challenges and stimulates you, then an opportunity in an organization that is computerizing its nursing documentation will be attractive. However, if people contact most appeals to you, such an environment may not be appropriate. If you like constant change and do not need to establish continuing relationships with clients, then emergency nursing may be an excellent career choice. You must articulate what excites you and makes you feel most alive and fulfilled.

### Recognizing Your Accomplishments

As you finish your self-assessment, you should be able to identify your strengths and limitations as well as your significant accomplishments over the past 5, 10, 15, or more years. The insights and answers to the "Who am I?" question can be found in each individual's personal and professional accomplishments. Accomplishments refer to those activities in which you went beyond what you were hired to do. They are not items on a job description. Rather they are situations in which you identified a challenge, used a specific approach, and had a successful outcome. Accomplishments do not need to be a big deal. But they do represent those times in your life that you made a difference. These accomplishments become the value added that you bring to any work environment. An accomplishment can be anything from being a member of your child's school's fundraising committee, to being elected as the unit representative on a committee, or to having an article published; it reflects those times in which you achieved a personal or professional best.

## CARLOTTA'S SELF-ASSESSMENT

My current position is staff nurse, Neonatal Intensive Care Unit (NICU). I graduated from a diploma nursing program, returned to school, and obtained a degree in nursing and then a certificate in neonatal nursing. I am very involved in two community groups: Big Sisters and my church. I have completed a very thorough self-assessment, and the following are some highlights from it. I especially value (1) autonomy—the personal freedom to set my own work schedule, (2) variety—of tasks and routines, and (3) team work—frequent interpersonal interactions. My "hard skills" include my clinical expertise in the care of neonates, and my "soft skills" include counselling and supporting families, problem solving in acute-care situations, and collaborating with others on the health care team in the NICU. I am also calm, decisive, flexible, and persuasive. I have an interest in people (particularly newborns) and things (including computer technology).

My personal accomplishments include being a Big Sister to a 12-year-old girl and being elected by my peers to my church pastoral committee. My professional accomplishments include identifying breast-feeding information needs of parents with babies in the NICU and designing a resource package for them. I also sit on our hospital Nurses' Week Committee and for the last 2 years have chaired the subcommittee on guest speakers. My strengths include my commitment to quality family-centred care, which is exhibited not only by my excellent nursing skills but also by my excellent communication and interpersonal skills with parents, whom I support while their child is in the NICU. My other strengths include my ability to work collaboratively with others in both my personal and professional life.

My current limitations include my reluctance to write and make presentations about the breast-feeding resource package I developed. Therefore I have identified two current skill gaps: public speaking and writing for professional journals.

## CONTINUING THE PROCESS

It is wise to use your journal to keep an ongoing record of all personal and professional experiences that have had an impact on your career. It is even better if you annotate this list (i.e., make personal notes about what you learned)—what you did or did not enjoy and why, and how you may wish to follow up on a particular interest or challenge. Your journal will become a working historical document that you can rely on to inform later decisions. Remember that your life experiences, values, self-knowledge, and goals will change over time. Not only may your work experience be varied and include different career opportunities within nursing, but your levels of expertise may broaden or become highly specialized. Over the years, you will also develop in many ways outside the professional arena. People's vocational interests change and grow, family commitments change (demanding more or less attention), and beliefs and values become clearer. Documenting such personal and professional history will provide you with an inventory of inner resources that will serve you well as you develop an ongoing career plan that will be realistic and fulfilling.

### Your Reality Check: Asking "How Am I Seen?"

Once you have completed your self-assessment, you must validate it. "How do others see me?" is the complementary and critical question you must now ask yourself. Careful career planning requires formal and informal feedback from managers, peers, friends, and family. You may derive this feedback from routine performance appraisals and from ongoing dialogue and discussion about your current performance and future possibilities. Asking for feedback is not easy, but successful career planning depends on your being open to new ideas and perspectives. It involves listening and accepting positive feedback and acknowledging the areas in which change is needed. Seeking advice about new skills that you may require and how to develop them also is essential.

Go back now and review again the accomplishments you identified in your journal and self-assessment. Now reflect on the feedback you have received about these achievements from your peers, manager, staff, friends, and family. Did anyone else know about what you considered an accomplishment? Nurses often have been hesitant to boast about what they have accomplished and how they have made a difference. It feels uncomfortable. Refer to Figure 3-2 to guide you in this process.

Getting feedback affirms where we shine. Before others can give us feedback, they need to know that we are open to hearing what will be said. Start with those individuals you trust. What three adjectives would they use to describe you both in and out of your workplace and why? What would they identify as your strengths and limitations? Now consider getting feedback from an individual whom you know, but not that well, and ask her or him the same questions. Asking such sources for feedback may be risky, but their responses will further enhance your self-assessment. You can also refer to any performance reviews, notes of appreciation, or personal notes you may have taken when you received feedback.

Think of how people have evaluated your strengths and limitations in the past. What have colleagues told you about your strengths, and what suggestions for improvement have they made? There may be many sources from which to validate your own self-assessment. Some regulatory bodies require self-assessment as part of quality assurance; the performance management program in your place of employment, including goal setting and performance appraisal, is another valuable resource. The evaluation component of projects, committees, and other activities may also provide some valuable information for you, and of course the informal comments of colleagues and friends are invaluable in helping you understand how you are seen by others.

You need a range of opinion to approximate the objective truth. No one welcomes criticism, but it can be instrumental in your career when it is delivered and received constructively and in the context of a caring relationship that encourages growth and self-development. For instance, you may hold an unrealistically high opinion of your attributes, which can lead to your setting your sights on a particular job or career goal and being continually disappointed at your lack of success. Alternatively, you may have an unrealistically low opinion of your attributes, which may prevent you from seeking

---

- Look at the accomplishments you identified in your self-assessment. What feedback did you get from your manager? Your peers? Others?
- What did these people say about your strengths and limitations?
- What three adjectives would these people use to describe you? Why?

---

Figure **3-2.** Completing your reality check.

positions well within your reach or lead to your selling yourself short in your current role. So be prepared to invite and listen carefully to feedback and to acknowledge those areas in yourself where change is needed. Ask for input about how to develop new skills and attitudes.

## CARLOTTA'S REALITY CHECK

To get feedback on my accomplishments, I developed a list of everyone who could possibly give me feedback. The list included the Executive Director, Big Sisters and my "little sister," the chair of the Pastoral Committee and three members of the committee, my nurse manager, the neonatologist, three of my peers, two families with whom I am currently working closely in the NICU, and the Chair of the Nurses' Week Committee. Out of this list, I chose five individuals, met with them, and asked them what three adjectives they would use to describe me and why. I was pleased with the responses, which included the following three strengths: I am caring (show concern for people), a creative problem solver (see many alternatives), and persistent (stick to tasks). Two individuals identified the same limitations—that I appear hesitant to speak in public about my accomplishments and that I have so much to offer but often my accomplishments go unnoticed.

## OTHER SELF-ASSESSMENT RESOURCES

At most times during your career, you will be able to complete the self-assessment and reality check on your own, using friends, family, and colleagues to help. However, there may be circumstances in which you require additional professional assistance. For example, you may have scanned your environment and completed your self-assessment and reality check but realize you are still quite confused and unclear about where your strengths lie and the nature of your limitations. Or you may believe that your environment is complex and that you are at a point in your career in which taking a different direction seems desirable, but you are not sure you have identified your own abilities and skills carefully enough to decide where to go. In such circumstances you may wish to consult a career counsellor and complete a more formal and comprehensive self-assessment. This can help you understand your attributes in a detailed manner and direct you to specific related career paths, which may diverge from or intersect with your current path.

If the services of a professional are required to complement your self-assessment, the counsellor can rely on a variety of well-researched and well-developed instruments to help you assess your strengths, traits, and characteristics objectively and relative to the work environment. It is helpful to familiarize yourself with the spectrum of assessment materials and then decide which ones to take and whom to entrust with the administration, scoring, feedback, and implementation of follow-up evaluation. Standardized tests in combination with your ongoing self-assessment may change your perceptions and open doors to new roles or settings within nursing or in alternate careers. Such standardized tests are designed to measure cognitive intelligence (e.g., Wechsler Adult Intelligence Scale-Revised [WAIS-R]), multiple intelligences (e.g., MI Inventory), emotional intelligence (e.g., EQ-i), personality (e.g., Myers-Briggs Type Indicator [MBTI]), interests (e.g., Campbell Interest and Skills Survey [CISS]), and lifestyle needs and values (e.g., Adult Balanced Life Enhancement Inventory [ABLE]). Tests that help you with career direction or understanding self include Career Occupational Preference System, Career Orientation Placement and Evaluation Survey, Career Exploration Inventory, and True Colors. Testing services may be available to you at no cost through an employee assistance program, the Internet, or at a career development centre associated with your workplace, a relocation or outplacement firm, your local university or community college, or the YM/YWCA. Do your research, secure references from satisfied clients, and select a professional who is a career development specialist.

## PUTTING IT ALL TOGETHER

Success and satisfaction depend on having the courage, confidence, and will to be authentic in your work. Self-assessment provides you with the means to do this. Whether you conduct a self-assessment independently or with the help of a professional career counsellor, you will be able to recognize and appreciate your full range of inner resources: intelligence, knowledge, skills, interests, personality, values, and motivations. The more research you do, the more thorough and realistic your findings will be. Your performance reviews and conversations with peers and managers with whom you have worked will serve as reality checks to deepen your self-knowledge. Take time to collect constructive feedback, and think it over carefully. Piece together all the data now to create a written, composite profile of your strengths and challenges. This document will serve as your passport to the new land of career research and enable you to negotiate the next three phases of the career planning and development process: creating your career vision, developing your strategic plan, and marketing yourself.

With an accurate sense of who you are and how others see you, you will be ready to explore job descriptions, physical and emotional environments, working conditions, and benefits to determine where you would have the most to contribute. Regularly revisiting your self-assessment will allow you to update your knowledge of self, set learning goals, develop career goals and action plans, and feel confident that you will love the work you do. Knowing your personal resources is a form of capital that represents an effective investment in your future. Use it and you will be the one who is in charge of your career, both now and in the future.

## REFERENCES

Crow, G.L. (2000). Knowing self. In Bower, F.L. (Ed.), *Nurses taking the lead: Personal qualities of effective leadership.* (pp. 15-37). Philadelphia: W.B. Saunders.
James-Neill, M. (1982). *The learning journal. NTL reading book for human relations training.* Arlington, VA: NTL Institute.
Maslow, A. (1970). *Motivation and personality* (2nd ed.). New York: Harper & Row.

## FURTHER READING

Bolles, R.N. (2002). *What color is your parachute? A practical manual for job-hunters & career changers.* Berkeley, CA: Ten Speed Press.
Bridges, W. (1997). *Creating you & co.* Reading, MA: Addison-Wesley.
Buckingham, M., & Clifton, D. (2001). *Now, discover your strengths.* New York: Simon & Schuster.
Covey, S. (1989). *The seven habits of highly effective people.* New York: Simon & Schuster.
Hafner, B. (2002). *Where do I go from here: Exploring your career alternatives within and beyond clinical nursing.* Philadelphia: J.B. Lippincott.
Moses, B. (1997). *Career intelligence: Mastering the new work and personal realities.* Toronto, Ontario, Canada: Stoddart.
Schein, E. (1990). *Discovering your real values* (2nd ed.). San Francisco: Pfeiffer & Co.

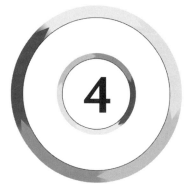

# Creating Your Career Vision

Mary M. Wheeler, RN, MEd

**Mary M. Wheeler** is a Partner in donnerwheeler, a consulting firm specializing in career planning and development within the health sector. Mary's consulting expertise is in career, organization, and human resource development, with a special interest in the human side of change. Mary is also a certified coach.

## Author Reflections

*My career visions, which have been shaped by all the attributes that make me who I am and what I want to be in this world, have taken me on journeys I never could have imagined when I began my nursing career. Having a vision keeps me looking ahead with anticipation and never looking back with regret.*

*The indispensable first step to getting the things you want in this life is this: decide what you want.*

**Ben Stein**

Vision is another word for a dream, an image of potentiality. More often than not we construct visions for our personal lives—the trip we dream about taking, the home we dream about purchasing, or the hopes we hold for our family's future—and then put plans in place to ensure that that dream is realized. Our dreams sustain us and keep us moving forward. Yet when it comes to our professional lives we often avoid or resist dreaming about what could be possible for our careers. Nurses need to create visions that describe where they want to go with their careers. They then need to develop action plans to ensure that the vision they create becomes a reality. These career visions sustain us as the health care environment continues to evolve.

In Chapters 2 and 3, we showed you how to use the first two phases of our career planning and development process, *Scanning Your Environment* and *Completing Your Self-Assessment and Reality Check*. These phases are fairly concrete. The third phase, *Creating Your Career Vision*, is somewhat more abstract, and its concepts may be harder to grasp. Creating a career vision is that point in the process where you integrate what you learned from your environmental scan with your self-assessment, and you begin to formulate an idea of what you want to do with your nursing career by taking a more active role in your career development. Where do you see yourself going? Do you like what you are currently doing, feel it is a good fit with your personal life, and want to develop within that role? Or have you learned that you enjoy change and variety and that it may be time to move on to other challenges? Because your vision of your potential future is grounded in your scan and self-assessment, it is focused on what is possible and realistic for you, both in the short-term and the long-term. Your career vision is the link between who you are and what you can become.

In this chapter you will learn about what is involved in the concept of career vision, why it is important to have one, and how to go about creating one of your own. In Chapter 5, Claire Mallette shows you how to set your short-term and long-term goals and how to develop a strategic plan to ensure that you reach those goals. Without career goals and a career plan, your vision will remain forever only a dream.

## WHAT IS A CAREER VISION?

A career vision is tempered by the realities of your environmental scan and self-assessment, but it is not determined by them. Those who have a career vision talk in terms of what is possible. They make use of all their resources, and they have the ability to harness and focus their energy. Having a career vision is perhaps the most forceful motivator for change that individuals can possess.

Dreaming is the beginning of all human endeavours. Unless you can dream, how do you know where you want to go? And until you know where you want to go, how can you sit down and plan how to get there? Dreams can be incredibly fragile, but individuals need to be encouraged to dream. You may say, "Why bother?" But if you do not, what could you be missing out on? How would you know your real potential? Lindaman and Lippitt (1979) point out that the choice is crucial, whether to cope reactively to a future created by others or to work creatively and strategically to craft a future you prefer. To shape that future, you must hold an image in your mind of what it is you really want. It is this use of imagination, whether initiated by idle dreaming or conscious intention, that will propel you into the future.

Remember back to when you chose nursing as a career. You formed some type of vision of what nursing would look like and what part you would play in it. You created that ideal vision for your work and your future. You had a purpose and a reason for being in which you envisioned a life filled with meaning and significance. McCarthy (1992) says that purpose is energy and that it is the single most motivating force there is. One needs a purpose, an answer to the question "Why do I exist?" before formulating a vision or a projection into the future. Purpose is a permanent, common thread woven throughout and in all parts of our lives. It exists in our past, present, and future.

Vision, on the other hand, is future based. It inspires because it paints a visual picture of where one is going by being on-purpose. Vision is a *where* question: "Where am I going with my purpose?" "Since purpose is the spark, then vision is the flame. It feeds the imagination, inspires the heart, and attracts others. Our vision is our dream and our hope. It sustains us during the inevitable trying times that come with choosing to live on-purpose" (McCarthy, 1992, p. 83). Over the years both you and the realities of the workplace may have undergone significant changes. Therefore you should be continuously reassessing whether that first picture still accurately depicts your current reality: Am I still feeling the way I felt when I chose nursing as a career, still doing what I want to be doing, still on-purpose?

Bridges (1994) encourages us to ask ourselves these two questions: What do I really want to do? What do I want so badly that I would do almost anything to achieve it? People who desire something discover talents they never knew they had. Because they believe in it, they argue their case so persuasively that they gain allies and solve problems that in any other setting would have been considered insoluble. They are passionate about their lives. When you are trying to decide what you are going to do next in your life, what you really desire is the only valid place to begin. Desire is the first and most important ingredient of the powerful motivation that is essential to career success.

In the future, success will rest on your adaptability, on your ability and commitment to embrace change, and on your assuming the active management of your own career. Change, although frightening and intimidating, can also be very rewarding. Embracing change means pushing yourself to explore all the possibilities, whether that is enriching your current work or looking for new opportunities inside or outside your workplace. Unless you take some risks, you will never really know the extent of your potential. The question no longer is "Can I change?" but rather "What type of change do I want?" That is what creating a career vision does; it answers the question, "What do I want?"

If you do not have some idea of what you want or where you want to go, you more often will just be reacting to events as they occur rather than choosing a direction in which to go. Nor will you easily be able to recognize and take advantage of an opportunity when it occurs. "Vision is important because it shows us where we are headed; it provides the insight, information and ideas about how to accomplish our goals; it gives us new direction; it helps us to make specific choices and decisions; it provides motivation and inspires us to keep going; it focuses us; it moves us toward what we want rather than what we do not want; it draws us forward and takes us beyond obstacles; and it gives meaning and purpose" (Bender, 1997, pp. 91-93). That is why having a career vision is crucial for nurses who want to have control over their career futures, whether they are staying where they are or making a change. A vision helps to guide our choices and direct our energy toward achieving our career goals. Many nurses have never considered that they can play a part in designing their career futures. Some may need to free themselves from a career path that others have expected of them before they can begin to formulate their own career vision. Other nurses will need to acknowledge that they have more choices than they had ever considered. These changes require a shift in orientation. You must move from being the observer about what "they" think you should be doing with your career to becoming an active participant in the picture—a goal setter, a doer. That means taking control of your career and your future, making choices, understanding the consequences, and moving forward.

Today, career success depends not only on having a dream but also on knowing how to turn that dream into a reality. Creating a career vision is the first step in that process. If followed by setting goals, developing a strategic plan, and marketing that plan, it can lead you to success, however you define it, for whatever may lie ahead.

## CREATING YOUR CAREER VISION

Wouldn't it be great to create your work the way you want it? You can, but first you need to create a vision for your work. It may be a more fulfilling version of what you are already doing, or it may be very different. Creating a career vision begins with taking time to do some active daydreaming about an ideal day in your future. Your career vision will be as individual as you are. Creating it will require you to ask yourself some important questions and give yourself permission to let go of what you previously thought possible. Sher (1983) asked, "Do you wake up every morning excited about the day ahead and delighted to be doing what you're doing, even if you're sometimes a little nervous and scared?" If not, what would make it that way for you? What is your fondest dream? Whatever it is, "As of right now I want you to start taking it very, very seriously!" (Sher, p. xi).

When you start, your vision doesn't need to be too realistic; that comes later in the process when you determine your options and set your career goals. Don't worry about your vision being too big, too vague, or too impossible. It should be grand and inspiring and, if it is an important dream, it may be a little scary. Hopkins (1986) says that when ancient mariners set off across uncharted waters to discover the lands of their dreams, their maps warned, "Here Be Dragons" (p. 10). If you want to pursue your dreams, you must be prepared to go where the dragons are. You should begin creating your career vision by believing that you can have your work be all that you envision. "How can I become the best I can be; how can I combine my skills and talents with my dreams?" With a clear career vision, a firm commitment, and the knowledge to bring it about, you will embark on a journey to discover your full potential.

### Try This

Find a quiet space where you will be undisturbed. Sit in a comfortable chair, and if you like, put on some relaxing music. Close your eyes so you can connect more easily with the music, your imagination, and creativity. When you are ready, record your responses to each of the following questions in a journal. As you learned in Chapter 3, journaling is an excellent way to have a conversation with yourself about how people, events, ideas, and feelings have made an impact on you and your career. As you move through the career planning and development process, keep your journal close at hand so you can jot down significant musings about career possibilities. After writing down your thoughts, read what you have written and then reflect on your writing.

Two key questions should guide you in the process of creating a career vision of your ideal work. The first question—**Where would I like to go?**—functions like a warm up or brainstorming session. Blue sky thinking is at work here; no answer is wrong. What have you always wanted, but not needed? In your journal start what McCarthy (1992) calls a want list, and what you can call a Career Want List. After you have exhausted listing all your dreams, start prioritizing them. If you had to choose between Number 1 and Number 2 on your list, which would you choose? If you had to choose between Number 3 and Number 4, which would you choose? And so on. You begin to formulate a draw sheet, similar to a scoring system used in sporting events. Keep going until you have two or three significant career wants. You have not eliminated the others, they have just become lower priorities. The second question—**What is my ideal vision for my work?**—provides more focus as you begin to create your career vision. As you answer this question, your evolving career vision should be influenced rather than determined by the data you gleaned from scanning your environment and completing your self-assessment. When you are ready, formulate your career vision in the present tense, as if it were occurring right now, and in as much descriptive detail as possible.

Remember that visioning is a creative process that helps us to translate our dreams into words or pictures that can be used to communicate that vision to others. Once you have a vision, start developing a picture. What does the vision look, feel, and sound like? Take some coloured markers and try to draw the vision. Post this in a prominent place and revisit it every time you pass by. Add to it and change it as new ideas emerge. Replay the vision in your head while you are waiting in line or doing tasks that do not require a lot of thought. Use your dream time to work on the vision. Before you go to sleep, tell yourself that you want to see your vision in your dreams and that you want to remember that vision when you get up. Keep your journal by your bed to record any thoughts as soon as you get up. Review examples of other people's visions that have been successful and check them against your vision (Bender, 1997).

As you create your career vision, reflect on what would it be like if it came to pass. What would be the advantages and disadvantages? Then consider what some possible scenarios would be if you did not move toward what you really wanted to do. Again ask yourself what would be the advantages and then the disadvantages of not pursuing your career vision. At this point you still have the ability to manoeuvre and to decide how comfortable the career vision feels. The first three phases of the career planning and development process begin to merge at this point, and by the time you set your career goals, your career vision should be grounded in reality.

## Self-Limiting Beliefs

The biggest barriers to creating a career vision are those we place on ourselves. As you moved through the process, did you come to the point where you said to yourself, "I want to (fill in your own career vision), but I can't because I'm too old, or I don't know how to go about applying for the position, or I'm not qualified?" Separate the real barriers (e.g., I'm not qualified) from the perceived ones (I'm too old). The real barriers can generally be overcome, but the perceived barriers or self-limiting beliefs will block us and our progress. They are the old entrenched beliefs that oppose a new idea. What we believe about ourselves and what could be possible are powerful determinants of our behaviour. That is why it is so important to explore our assumptions and clarify the values that underpin them.

Pay attention to these self-limiting beliefs, because they have the potential to inhibit your ability to create what you want. In your journal, list some self-limiting beliefs that could prevent you from doing what you really want to do. Now go back to Chapter 3, review your self-assessment, and reflect on your strengths; these are your enablers, and these will provide the evidence that you can do what you want to do. Your strengths will probably outweigh your self-limiting beliefs. Many defeat their desires because they concentrate on why "I can't" rather than why "I can." Schwartz (1959) says that "when you believe something is impossible, your mind goes to work for you to prove why, but when you believe, really believe, that something can be done, your mind goes to work for you and helps you find the ways to do it" (p. 85).

There are situations in which the environmental constraints or real barriers such as funding, employer policies, or education may affect your achieving your career vision. Once again use the skills you learned in Chapter 2 to scan your environment, become aware of those constraints, and put a plan in place to deal with them. Even with these supposed environmental constraints, Gladwell (2000) says that the world around us "may seem like an immovable, implacable place. It is not. With the slightest push—in just the right place—it can be tipped" (p. 259). If you are always walking away from your dreams, it may be that you are afraid you will fail or, worse, that you will succeed. If you are afraid of something, try to understand what it is and why it scares you and then take action to overcome it. Action cures fear. Until you confront your fears your dreams will never be as big as they possibly could be. You must believe in your potential and yourself. The power of positive thinking cannot be underestimated. Think big!

## What Is It You Want to Create?

According to Gershon and Straub (1989), what we believe is what we create. We must clear our self-limiting beliefs before we can realize new beliefs. To realize new beliefs, we must have a clear vision of what we want to create. They suggest using three techniques: (1) affirmation, or creating a statement of what we want to create in our life; (2) visualization, or forming a mental picture or image of what we want to create; and (3) germination, or the energizing process, that is, being committed to a vision we believe will occur and doing what it takes to make it happen. Talbot (1994) builds on the visualization step and suggests that individuals pretend it is a year from today and they have become very successful (however they define successful). Visualize this success; make a picture, and describe it. Then describe the steps that were taken to get there. Once your career vision is written down, say it out loud. What does it sound like? Would you be prepared to share it with others? When you feel comfortable sharing your career vision, your network enlarges and the probability of success increases. How can anyone help you if you do not let them know what you want? You need both to articulate and to own your career vision.

Meghan is a staff nurse currently working in labour and delivery at an acute care teaching hospital. She loves her job and has no intention to leave her unit at this time; however, she would like to enrich her practice while staying in place. When she scanned her external environment, two important trends presented themselves: the focus on family-centred care and the challenge of providing continuity of care for mothers and babies that has resulted from shorter hospital stays. Meghan observed that many of these mothers were returning to the emergency department shortly after discharge with complaints of their infants' failure to thrive and dehydration. When Meghan completed her self-assessment, she recognized that she not only has expert clinical and people skills but also that she values responsibility, the opportunity to influence others, and working as part of a team. She also identified a limitation: she does not have enough experience with patient education. Meghan's ideal vision for her work looks like this:

I am working on a maternal child unit providing educational services for new mothers and babies. I work with members of a team who are striving to reduce the frequency in which mothers and their babies return to hospital after discharge.

Yael works as a clinical nurse specialist in psychiatry at a community hospital. When she scanned her environment, she saw that, as a result of hospital restructuring, a new position was opening up for a nurse manager who would be responsible for a three-site combined psychiatric services program. Before her current position, Yael had filled the role of nurse manager on her unit for 7 months while the incumbent was on maternity leave. When Yael completed her self-assessment, she realized that she not only liked the role and the responsibilities of being the interim nurse manager, but also she received positive feedback from colleagues, particularly about her supportive relationship with staff on the unit and her leadership in the development of a psychiatric community focus group. She also identified a limitation: her management experience was only hands on. She had limited formal management education, particularly in the area of financial planning. Yael's ideal vision for her work looks something like this:

> I am a nurse manager, providing strategic direction for the development of the new programs in psychiatry at the regional level. I am coaching staff in their new roles as direct service providers and am working as a valuable member of the newly appointed regional senior management team.

Caitlin was teaching oncology nursing full-time in a university nursing program. Six months ago she took an academic administrative position, which decreased her teaching load but increased her broader departmental responsibilities. Caitlin has two young children. After completing her self-assessment, particularly in the beliefs and values component, she acknowledged that she is unhappy and unable to manage her workload and still maintain a healthy family life with two young children at home. She also acknowledged that her passion is teaching, not management. Her greatest joy comes from spending time with her children and from working with nursing students and helping them realize their potential. Caitlin's ideal vision for her work looks like this:

> I have relinquished my administrative responsibilities and I am now teaching part-time. I have more time and energy for both my children and my students.

All three nurses put their dreams into words. Your dream can help you create your future, whether that is doing what you are currently doing or looking for new possibilities. Your dream is your guide.

## Determining the Options

Now that you are able to describe your ideal career vision, it is time to determine possible career options. Determining your career options involves recognizing what may be feasible, clarifying your choices, and making decisions. It is the process of reality testing in which you now ask yourself, "How realistic is my career vision?" As Levoy (1997) asks, "Is this a vision I'm meant to fulfill or just a grandiose fantasy?" (p. 44). Every vision is realistic depending on how much time, patience, and energy you want to put into achieving it. Intuitively we will know when our dreams are unrealistic because we have limited time, patience, and energy to commit to them.

Determining your options is a short but crucial step. It is done just after you create your career vision but just before you set your career goals. These choices or options emerge from the congruence between your environmental scan and your self-assessment. When you were creating your career vision, you kept the information in your scan and self-assessment somewhat in the background so that you did not risk being inhibited and not daring to dream. Now that you have your vision and are determining your career options, the data from your scan and self-assessment should become more influential and assume a place in the foreground of your mind. Which options are viable will vary with changes in the work climate and in yourself, so remember to continually scan your environment and update your self-assessment.

> Meghan's career vision for herself is to provide some form of comprehensive patient education to new mothers. One environmental constraint is that no additional funding is available to increase education programs to new mothers. Meghan will need to decide how realistic this vision is for her career satisfaction and how much effort she wants to put into seeing her vision realized: what is possible and realistic for the short term, and what should be planned for the longer term. For example, in the short term Meghan could consult with others on the team regarding the latest evidence on the cost-effectiveness of educational programs as part of a strategy to influence management related to the efficacy and efficiency of educational services to new mothers.

Your career vision may be a confirmation that you are already doing what you love, or it may be a revelation of an entirely new way to think about expressing yourself in your work. You are more likely to attain satisfying work when you follow your personal passions, pursue your interests, and utilize your strengths. Go back to scanning your environment and your self-assessment. Does your career vision fit with what the new world of work requires and with the skills, talents, and abilities you have to offer? If so, then you now have a vision of what you want to build, and you can move forward as fast or as slowly as you desire. If not, you have not wasted your time. Review your scan, your self-assessment, and your career vision. If it still appears realistic, the timing may just not be right. Don't let go of the vision; be patient yet persistent. Make adjustments so that you are positioned to take advantage of better circumstances when the climate changes and the opportunities arise. Surround yourself with those who will support and encourage you when your career vision appears impossible.

## CONCLUSION

Now that you have articulated your dream, you are ready to make plans to move toward that vision for your career. You know what is around you, you know yourself, and you have your dream. Chapter 5, "Developing Your Strategic Career Plan," will explain in more detail how to accomplish this next phase in the career planning and development process. This next phase will help you answer the question, "How will I get there from here?" It will provide you with strategies to close the gap between vision and reality. These strategies include setting clear goals that will convert your dream from a vague concept into an action-oriented goal statement from which you can design your strategic career plan. Go for it!

## REFERENCES

Bender, P.U. (1997). *Leadership from within.* Toronto, Ontatio, Canada: Stoddart.

Bridges, W. (1994). *JobShift: How to prosper in a workplace without jobs.* Reading, MA: Addison-Wesley.

Gershon, D., & Straub, G. (1989). *Empowerment: The art of creating your life as you want it.* New York: Dell.

Gladwell, M. (2000). *The tipping point: How little things can make a big difference.* Boston: Little, Brown.

Hopkins, W. (1986). *A goal is a dream taken seriously.* King of Prussia, PA: The HRD Quarterly.

Levoy, G. (1997). *Callings: Finding and following an authentic life.* New York: Three Rivers Press.

Lindaman, E., & Lippitt, R. (1979). *Choosing the future you prefer.* Washington, DC: Development Publications.

McCarthy, K. (1992). *The on-purpose person.* Colorado Springs, CO: Pinon Press.

Schwartz, D. (1959). *The magic of thinking big.* New York: Simon & Schuster.

Sher, B. (1983). *Wishcraft: How to get what you really want.* New York: Ballantine Books.

Talbot, D. (1994, August 16). A break from the huddle. *The Globe and Mail,* p. B20.

## FURTHER READING

Edwards, P., & Edwards, S. (1996). *Finding your perfect work: The new career guide to making a living, creating your life.* New York: J.P. Tarcher.

Edwards, P., & Edwards, S. (2000). *The practical dreamers handbook.* New York: Putnam.

Haldane, B. (1996). *Career satisfaction and success: A guide to job and personal freedom.* Indianapolis, IN: JIST Works.

Jarow, R. (1995). *Creating the work you love.* Rochester, VT: Destiny Books.

Jones, L. (1996). *The path: Creating your mission statement for work and life.* New York: Hyperion.

Sher, B. (1994). *I could do anything if I only knew what it was.* New York: Dell.

Sinetar, M. (1987). *Do what you love and the money will follow.* New York: Dell.

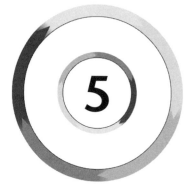

# Developing Your Strategic Career Plan

Claire Mallette, RN, MSc, PhD (cand.)

**Claire Mallette** is the Chief Nursing Officer and Director of Professional Practice at the Workplace Safety and Insurance Board in Ontario and a PhD candidate in the Faculty of Nursing, University of Toronto. Her areas of expertise are in organizational behaviour focusing on the psychological contract, employment relationships, quality work environments, and the issue of retention and recruitment.

▌Author Reflections

*Throughout my career, having a strategic career plan has helped guide my decisions to what the next step should be to achieve my career goals. My plan has given me the courage to take risks, face my fears, as well as recognize and seize the opportunities destiny has provided me.*

*Chance favours the prepared mind.*

**Louis Pasteur**

## WHAT IS A CAREER PLAN?

In *Alice in Wonderland*, Alice was confronted with which direction to take. She turned to the Cheshire Cat and asked, "Would you tell me, please, which way I ought to walk from here? The Cheshire Cat responded, "That depends a good deal on where you want to get to." Planning one's career very much depends a good deal on where you want to "get to." Although chance occurrences may play a role in shaping your career, planning and preparation put you in a position to take full advantage of chance occurrences, to recognize opportunity, and to assess risk.

In the previous chapters you identified where you want to go by scanning the environment, completing a self-assessment, and creating your career vision. This chapter explores the actual plan for attaining your vision. Career planning is a lifelong process of looking ahead and making decisions of what to do next. A career plan consists of the identification of goals, action steps, resources, timelines, and evaluation of success. Many similarities can be drawn between the nursing process and your career plan. You create your vision and identify goals by assessing your inner feelings and dreams and the environment. Once you have identified your long- and short-term goals, you need to develop an action plan.

By creating a plan, you begin to move and to make decisions. Each decision builds on previous decisions and leads to action. Each action then affects the choices you will have in the future. A strategic career plan and clearly defined goals will enable you to build on options that guide you in achieving your vision. Finally, as in the nursing process, it is important to evaluate whether you achieved the desired goals. As you proceed, the incremental steps you take to achieve your goals will become recognizable and, when reached, will provide you with additional incentives to persevere with your strategic career plan. A career is a lifelong investment and, as with any investment, planning pays off! In this chapter you will learn how to create your own career plan and how to implement it.

## ISSUES IN DEVELOPING YOUR PLAN

### Taking Risks

To have a successful career action plan, you will need to take risks. When you create your own future, there will always be risks. Look at individuals whom you consider to be successful. Do you think they took risks to get there? Absolutely! Did you know that you have a risk muscle that without exercise will waste away (Von Oech, 1986)? Exercise your risk muscle. In your professional life, there is neither growth nor gain without risk. In fact, your greatest risk lies in not pursuing your future, in not advancing into the unknown, and in not trying to reach your full potential (White, 1990). Risk is part of career advancement (Foord Kirk, 1996). To assess your readiness for taking risks, Simonsen (2000) outlines several questions you can ask yourself, which are listed in the box below.

---

**Readiness for Risk Taking**

- How have you responded to new situations in the past?
- How do you approach new or difficult situations?
- How do you identify risk?
- How do you decrease the risk when you embark on new challenges?
- Have you ever found yourself paralyzed by the fear of the undesired results?
- Do you ever act impulsively without concern for the outcome?

---

The answers to these questions will provide you with insight into your risk-taking potential and how to manage it to the best of your abilities. The first step in managing risk is to assess the level of it. This can be achieved by understanding what you can and cannot control and by being realistic about what you can and cannot achieve (Helfand, 1999). Then identify the worst-case and best-case scenarios and ask yourself whether you are willing to accept the consequences. Focus on the challenge instead of fearing it, and learn to expect change rather than dreading it. By embracing change, you will learn how to manage risk (Foord Kirk, 1996). "What is the worst thing that could happen if I do this?" can be a very useful question to ask yourself.

## Setting Career Goals

The first step in career planning is to make a decision, even if it is a tentative one, about a career goal. In previous chapters, you answered questions related to where you would like to go and your ideal vision for your work. What was it you wanted to change or accomplish? If you do not set goals, your career vision will forever remain only a dream. Change and growth take you into uncharted territories and can create fear and uncertainty. Goal setting can help you to move beyond your fear and anxiety by establishing sound planning and taking smart, calculated risks. Your success in whatever you choose to do depends on your ability to set goals.

A goal is the purpose or objective toward which an endeavour is directed. It keeps you looking toward the future, focused on finishing, on doing it all, and on doing it right. Choosing and setting goals means you are serious about taking charge of your career. When setting goals, it is important to remember that a goal is a concrete action or event. It is a matter of facts, not feelings.

### Types of Career Goals

There are a variety of career goals. Simonsen (2000) outlines the different types of career goals you can have depending on what you want to achieve. For example, everyone should have *development goals*. These types of goals result in personal growth. *Role enhancement goals* are those you need when you strive for a different stage in your career. Examples of these goals are looking for a new position or expanding your current role. When you have identified that your present organization is no longer conducive to your career vision, you will want to set *external move goals*. These goals involve looking for career opportunities outside of the organization; although this process can be anxiety provoking, it can lead you in new and exciting directions. Another new career direction is the decision to change your career field. If you are dissatisfied with your career or your interests are in one area but your work is in another, you may decide to make some *career changing goals*. These might involve leaving your current profession of nursing and seeking another career. *Lifestyle goals* are related to the work/life balance that you want to achieve. You may decide you want to decrease the amount of time you are working as you head toward retirement. This would involve setting goals to take less responsibility or to take a part-time job. Depending on where you are in your career, any of these goals can lead you toward increased satisfaction in your professional development and personal well-being.

### CHAPTER 5

### Criteria for Goal Setting

Your answers to your vision questions are the beginnings of setting your long-term and short-term goals. Setting the long-term goal is the first step.

> Magdalen's long-term goal on graduation with a BScN was that she wanted to be a Chief Nurse Executive (CNE) by the time she reached 45 years of age.

Although this is a good long-term goal, it can seem overwhelming. The way to get beyond this feeling is to break down the long-term goal into short-term goals. If the short-term goals still seem overwhelming, break them down even more until you have a set of comfortable steps that lead you toward your future career. Short-term goals help you to keep the momentum needed to achieve your career plan (Alberta Advanced Education and Career Development, 1999).

> For Magdalen to achieve her goal, she broke down her long-term goal in her career plan into short-term goals. She knew she would need to go back to school and get a master's degree, possibly even a PhD, and gain experience in leadership positions. She broke down the leadership positions even more by identifying that she first needed to be a team leader, then a manager, and then a program director.

When setting your goals, you need to make sure they are achievable, realistic, specific, and measurable; have a timeline attached; and are supported by those who will be directly affected by your decision, including partners, family, colleagues, and friends. Without following this strategy, the goals will be vague, and it will be difficult to identify how to reach them.

Is the goal achievable and realistic? If it is not realistic, then you are setting yourself up for failure. Magdalen's goal of being a CNE would be unrealistic if she wanted to achieve this immediately after completing her undergraduate nursing program. Goals need to be specific. If they are not specific, then it is difficult to identify an action plan to achieve the goal. An example of a vague goal is "I want to nurse at a more advanced level." Although the dream and long-term goal have been identified, this type of goal does not set the plan into action. To do this, you need to make the goal more specific.

> Jiao wanted to be an advanced practice nurse. A specific long-term goal for her would be the following: "My long-term goal is to become a Clinical Nurse Specialist in Pediatrics within the next 5 years." To achieve this goal she needs to break it down into smaller goals.
>
> Within the next 2 months, I will:
>
> - Find out more about the role
> - Explore the necessary qualifications to achieve this goal
>
> Within the next 6 months, I will:
>
> - Identify universities that offer the necessary courses
> - Begin the application process well ahead of the deadline for application submission

By making your goals so specific, you are able to clearly identify and commit to beginning to make your career plan a reality.

You may choose a combination of short-term and long-term goals to transform your career vision into a reality. Moreover, you can concentrate on one goal at a time, pursue two at once, or balance a short-term and a long-term goal. Pursuing multiple goals encourages flexibility. It helps you feel more in control and less at the mercy of external forces (e.g., organizational change) so you have other options from which to choose if your desired direction becomes blocked.

Timelines and indicators of success are important to articulate in order to help you target your activities and stay focused. Timelines help you stay motivated, particularly for long-term goals (Simonsen, 2000). We often resist setting timelines for fear of not being able to meet them. However, timelines ensure that you dedicate your time and resources to accomplish the assigned goals. To set your timelines, ask yourself how much time you will need to achieve your goal.

When you accomplish your goals within the timelines, celebrate! It is important to recognize and reward yourself for your successes. If you do not achieve your goal within the designated timeline, examine why this occurred. Was the timeline unrealistic? Were there changes in the environment that you could not control? Once you have examined the reasons why the goal was not achieved, you can set yourself another target date or intentionally stop trying to achieve the goal. As Sher (1983) points out, sometimes there is no way to find out whether or not a particular goal really suits you except by trying it. If it does not suit you, you have still gained something priceless—the experience of making real progress toward a goal and the practical skills for doing it. These are skills that can be applied to achieving any goal.

A goal should move you from the intangible to the tangible. The clearer you are about your goals, the easier it will be to develop a plan of action. Remember that career goals should be realistic (I can do it), desirable (I want to do it), and motivating (I will work to make it happen). Be prepared to keep reevaluating and possibly altering your career goals to achieve your career vision. Setting clear goals involves converting your dream from a vague concept into an action-oriented goal statement from which you can design your strategic career plan.

### *Moving in Different Career Directions to Achieve Your Goals*

Just as your career plan may involve working on several complementary goals at once, so too should you consider moving in a variety of career directions to take the most effective action steps toward those goals. Career directions, or the avenues or pathways you travel on to reach your career vision, exist both within and between organizations. Kaye (1993) coined the phrase, "up is not the only way," (p. 26) because she foresaw a changing business environment in which people need to pursue development not as a ladder upward but instead in terms of a variety of moves. In today's health care climate, restructuring is creating flatter organizations with even fewer rungs on the ladder to the top. Kaye argued for a shift in perceiving career success from a vertical paradigm to a new, multidirectional paradigm, or from a ladder to a lattice. There are several career directions you can choose—lateral (moving sideways), vertical (moving up), or realignment (moving down or out). You can also choose to remain where you are and enhance your current role or position through a number of professional and personal activities.

*Lateral: Moving Sideways.* In a lateral move you seek out a new position but stay at the same level of responsibility. Nurses often choose this type of move when they want to remain at the bedside but seek new challenges and learning opportunities. Moving in a lateral career direction is a great way to not only increase your knowledge level and experience but also to recharge your batteries through renewed job satisfaction.

> Neil wanted to stay at the front line yet have new challenges. He achieved this goal by transferring from an orthopaedic surgical unit to the operating room.

Nurses also choose a lateral move to increase their knowledge, skills, and experience to help them reach their long-term goal.

Sometimes, however, you are not the one who initiates the lateral move. Some organizations routinely rotate staff laterally to keep them challenged and increase their employability skills. An organization may move you laterally because of restructuring or because your current position has become redundant. If you are in a unionized workplace, your union seniority may allow you to move laterally and "bump" another nurse with less seniority. Regardless of the reason for the lateral move, always look at it as a way to grow and increase your skills. In many situations your employer will provide continuing education to help you make the transition to the new position. Take advantage of the situation and build your repertoire of new skills.

*Vertical: Moving Up.* Your self-assessment may tell you that you have the ability and motivation to assume more responsibility and that a vertical move is appropriate for you. Although the flattening of organizations has resulted in fewer available leadership positions, there are always some opportunities for moving up in an organization. Traditionally, this meant being employed by one employer for your entire career and moving up the corporate ladder over time. In today's work environment, however, you may need to consider moving to another organization when a plateau in your career has been reached.

To achieve your vision, you need to scan the environment within your present organization and other organizations to identify both the organization's needs and your potential contributions. If there is congruence between the two, then a vertical move may be the right decision.

> Magdalen, whose long-term goal was to become a CNE, moved vertically to achieve her goal of obtaining a senior management position. To achieve this goal, she did a successful scan of her own and other organizations to identify the availability of leadership positions. She found no available positions

in her present organization and therefore decided to move to another organization to facilitate reaching her ultimate vision.

*Realignment: Moving Down.* Nurses often balance multiple demands such as pursuing a career, raising children, going to school, and taking care of aging parents. As a result, nurses are now making career choices related to work-life balance. They are demanding that work be a part of their lives—not all of it (Simonsen, 2000). For some, moving down is a way to move forward. There are many ways to achieve this. One method is taking a position with less responsibility. Other ways are through job sharing or part-time work. These can be good ways of achieving work-life balance for nurses with family responsibilities. For the more mature nurse, moving down to a part-time position can be a good way to achieve balance between having a career and starting to prepare for retirement.

> Deborah is 52, works full-time, and wants to continue to work in the emergency unit. However, she is finding the 12-hour and night shifts difficult to manage with the needs of her aging mother, who has moved in to live with her and her family. She would like to continue her nursing career and determines that working part-time is the best option for her.

*Realignment: Moving Out.* For some nurses, continuing to be a nurse is not in their career vision. They would like to leave the profession and start a new career. Changing a career mid-life or beyond is becoming more common as a result of events such as jobs ending or early retirement packages. For others, their interests lie in a new area and they want to leave the profession to seek out new learning opportunities and challenges. Regardless of the reasons for leaving nursing, it is important to recognize that you have developed many transferable skills during your nursing career. To identify these skills, review your self-assessment to determine which of them will best help you to move on a new career path.

## Developing an Action Plan

Once you have identified and written down your goals, you are ready to make an action plan. An action plan provides you with the answer to the question, "How do I achieve my goals?" A plan is like a map outlining a series of specific goal-directed activities that over time will guide you to your destination. You are taking control of your future by writing down the specific strategies required to achieve your goals. By having a well-developed action plan, you will be able to recognize and take advantage of career opportunities when they occur. Without a plan, long-term career goals may appear unattainable or become unattainable. Although it may take time to achieve your vision, the plan helps to ensure that you are continually working in the desired direction.

### When Should I Start My Career Plan?

You should begin your career plan as soon as you have created your career vision, determined your options, and set your goals. As you learned in the previous chapter, your options will change throughout your career. Having a plan ensures that you will be able to build on options that are best suited to achieving your vision. Getting started signals your commitment to acting on a specific goal. It indicates that you are serious about embarking on the journey toward your overall vision and that you are ready to address each of the components of an effective plan.

### What Goes into the Plan?

A career action plan includes identifying goals, action steps, timelines, and indicators of success. To create this plan, you will need some dedicated time, energy, and creativity. Do not worry if your plan is not perfect. It will be a work in progress. The only way your plan will remain useful to you is if you continually assess whether it reflects what you want to achieve in light of changes in your environmental scan, self-assessment, and career stage. Your indicators of success will help you to evaluate your plan at different stages in your career.

It is important to write down your action plan. Without a written version, it is easy to forget steps or fall out of sequence with the things that need to be achieved. A written plan also makes it much easier to continually review, refine, and re-evaluate both your goals and your progress. See Figure 5-1 for Magdalen's Career Plan.

A career plan is more effective when it is broken down into specific manageable action steps. These steps form building blocks toward achieving well-defined goals. Action steps also help you track your progress and are tangible evidence that you are moving in the right direction to reach your goal. To identify your action steps complete the following sentence: "To achieve this goal, I will...." It is important to identify what experiences will help you achieve each action step and what financial commitment will be required.

> Sheila had the long-term goal to work in public health within 3 years of graduating from her undergraduate program. She began to meet her long-term goal by setting the short-term goal of learning more about the community and about public health nursing. She wrote out her action steps as follows: "To achieve this goal, I will learn more about the role by reading the nursing and public health literature, going on the Internet to learn about different positions, and talking to people who are working in public health. I will do this in the next 3 months."

### Identifying Your Resources

The most effective career plans are not developed in isolation. Once you have decided on your career plan, it is important to examine the resources and opportunities within your environment that you can take advantage of. Many resources are available to you. You can access information from the Internet, newspaper, professional publications, professional organizations, a career center, workshops, your network, and your mentors. Making a

*Text continued on p. 58*

**Magdalen's Vision:** To provide leadership in nursing and health care in the hospital setting.
**Long-Term Goal:** I will be a Chief Nurse Executive before I reach age 45.

| Short-Term Goals | Action Steps and Timelines | Resources | Indicators of Success |
|---|---|---|---|
| I will work as a front-line nurse on a surgical or medical unit in an acute care setting for 3 to 5 years | In order to achieve this goal I will:<br>• Update my résumé in the next 3 weeks.<br>• Identify resources that can assist me in identifying hospitals with full-time positions within the next 2 weeks.<br>• Identify acute care hospitals that have full-time positions available within the next month.<br>• Contact both the Nursing and Human Resources Departments within the next month.<br>• Send them my résumé within the next 6 weeks.<br>• Prepare for the interview process. | • Internet<br>• Newspaper advertisements<br>• Peers who have recently graduated<br>• Nursing and Human Resources Departments within organizations | • I have a front-line nursing position in an acute care hospital. |

| | | | |
|---|---|---|---|
| While working as a front-line nurse, I will become involved in leadership activities. | In order to achieve this goal I will: <br> • Seek out mentors by establishing relationships upon entering the organization. <br> • Volunteer to be involved in nursing initiatives both on the unit and hospital-wide by volunteering for a unit-based project within the first year and a hospital-based initiative within 2 years. <br> • Begin to develop my leadership portfolio by becoming involved in my professional association and attending meetings. | • Colleagues <br> • Professors from my undergraduate program <br> • Supervisors <br> • Hospital communications | • I am a team leader on my unit. <br> • I regularly attend chapter meetings in my professional association. |

*Continued*

Figure **5-1.** Magdalen's career plan.

| Short-Term Goals | Action Steps and Timelines | Resources | Indicators of Success |
|---|---|---|---|
| In approximately 5 years, I will return to school part-time to obtain my Masters in Nursing degree (focusing on nursing administration) and will complete the program within 3 to 4 years. | In order to achieve this goal I will:<br>• Begin to identify appropriate universities and programs by dialoguing with my network and by doing Internet searches when I have worked in my front-line positions for 3½ years.<br>• Begin the application process 3 months before the application deadline. This includes having a colleague read my letter of intent.<br>• Continue to seek out leadership opportunities within my organization as I go to school.<br>• Expand my network by establishing relationships with peers and professors in the School of Nursing.<br>• Run for an elected position within my professional organization 2 years into my studies. | • Internet<br>• Colleagues<br>• Friends<br>• Resource people at the universities<br>• Funding opportunities<br>• Peer-reviewed journals | • I have a Masters in Nursing Administration.<br>• I am a regional representative for my professional association.<br>• I have a mentor from the Administration program at the School of Nursing. |

| | | |
|---|---|---|
| On completion of my Master's program, I will obtain a leadership position (such as Unit Manager) and will work in this position for approximately 3 to 5 years. | In order to achieve this goal I will:<br>• Scan the environment for leadership opportunities within my organization and in other organizations 6 months before graduation.<br>• Develop my leadership knowledge, skills, and abilities by dialoguing with mentors on an ongoing basis.<br>• Take on a leadership role for a hospital-wide initiative within the first 2 years.<br>• Continue to have a leadership role within my professional organization. | • Supervisors within my organization<br>• Colleagues<br>• Mentors<br>• Internet<br>• Newspaper advertisements<br>• Books and peer-reviewed journals | • I am a unit manager. |

Figure **5-1**, cont'd For legend, see p. 53.

*Continued*

| Short-Term Goals | Action Steps and Timelines | Resources | Indicators of Success |
|---|---|---|---|
| I will seek out further education in leadership and administration by completing an executive leadership program. | In order to achieve this goal I will:<br>• Identify appropriate universities and programs by dialoguing with my network and by doing Internet searches 6 months before the application process.<br>• Identify the program where I want to apply, as well as the requirements and costs.<br>• Obtain financial resources to cover travel, leave of absence from work, child care arrangements, and tuition fees.<br>• Begin the application process 4 to 6 months before the application deadline. | • Supervisors<br>• Funding agencies<br>• Internet<br>• Colleagues<br>• Professors<br>• Mentors | • I am enrolled in the Executive Leadership Post-Master's Certificate program at the Business School. |

On completion of the executive leadership program, I will obtain a senior management level position (such as Program Director within an organization) while continuing to develop a portfolio and obtain the necessary knowledge, skills, and abilities to become a CNE. This will be achieved within the next 5 to 7 years.

In order to achieve this goal I will:
- Begin to scan and use my network to identify opportunities for senior management positions 6 months before graduation.
- After graduation, become actively involved in policy development within my organization and for the nursing community at large by sitting on government task forces within 3 years.
- Assume a senior leadership position such as Vice President or President of my professional organization within the next 2 to 3 years.
- Continue to seek support through ongoing dialogue with mentors.
- Continue to scan the environment and be alert to opportunities to become a CNE.

- Colleagues
- Mentors
- Internet
- Newspaper advertisements
- Nursing and Human Resource Departments within organizations

- I am my hospital's representative on the regional health planning council.
- I am a Program Director and am actively seeking CNE positions in a variety of settings.

Figure **5-1**, cont'd For legend, see p. 53.

thoughtful inventory of your available and potential resources should be your first step in creating the action steps associated with each of your goals. Start by asking yourself the questions listed in the box below.

### Resource Inventory

**Whom Should I Talk To?**

- Who do I know in a similar role?
- Who has been helpful as a mentor in the past?
- Whom should I approach to be a mentor?
- Whom do I want to meet?

**What Should I Read?**

- Where can I look for information that I need to carry out the actions within my plan?
- How can I ensure that I keep up-to-date on what is going on in the world around me?

**Where Should I Spend Some Time?**

- What experiences will help me complete each action step?

**What Do I Need to Invest?**

- How much time will each action step demand?
- What financial commitment does my plan require?

Making a thoughtful inventory of your available and potential resources is the first step you should take to begin implementing the action steps associated with each of your goals.

Magdalen, whose ultimate goal was to become a CNE, had a short-term goal to develop advanced leadership skills. To achieve this goal, she planned the action step of completing an intensive executive leadership program. She identified that completing this course would require financial resources to cover travel, a leave of absence from work, child care arrangements, and the program fee. Knowing this information in advance permitted her to make the appropriate plan that considered the necessary resources.

The Internet is a valuable resource that can assist you in doing your research as you develop your career plan. By using a search engine (e.g., www.google. com) you can access thousands of organizations, available positions, and required qualifications.

The people you know and even those you do not know can be very valuable in giving you feedback and suggestions about your career plan and job search. Chapter 6 discusses the importance of networking in more depth.

### Assessing and Evaluating Plans and Goals

*Indicators of Success.* How will you know that your plan is working? If you have identified your long-term and short-term goals and documented your plan, including specific action steps, required resources, and timelines, you have a good start at identifying measures of success. Think about what you hope to accomplish with your plan. Completing a specific action step that clearly moves you toward a goal may be one indication of a workable plan. Assessing that you are professionally stimulated and happy doing what you are doing at a particular point in time may be another indicator of a successful career plan. Another sign of a good plan may be feeling that you have successfully taken charge of your own career. As you design your own plan, think about what success will look like for you. You also may define success differently at various stages in your career. Record your personal indicators to help you evaluate your plan at those different stages. See pp. 52 to 57 for Magdalen's career plan.

## HOW DO I KEEP MY PLAN WORKING FOR ME?

Career plans should be dynamic, responsive to personal circumstances, and professionally stimulating. To ensure that your plan remains flexible and relevant to your career vision, you must continuously re-evaluate your goals and your means of reaching them. You should be ready to adjust your plan as aspects of your self-assessment change, as your continuously updated environmental scan indicates that significant changes have occurred around you, or as you move into different stages of your career. Having a well-developed strategic career plan will also enable you to recognize and take advantage of career opportunities as they occur.

Magdalen, who aspired to be a hospital CNE, developed a detailed plan with concrete goals and action steps. As a result, she was able to seize opportunities of moving vertically toward her vision. As a series of circumstances arose, she advanced from a director of nursing position and from completing an executive leadership course to becoming president of a professional organization, the chair of a provincial task force, and finally a Chief Nurse Executive.

John thought he might like to work with older adults and had a short-term goal of finding a position that would let him "try it out." He accepted a casual position in a nursing home, which confirmed his interest in gerontology, gave him opportunities to gain experience and credibility as a practitioner, and eventually led to his being asked to consider a full-time position. Continual self-assessment helped John to refine his plan and develop a concrete goal related to securing a full-time position working with older adults.

## WHAT WILL YOU DO IF YOU LOSE YOUR JOB TOMORROW? DO YOU HAVE A PLAN?

Times have changed, and losing one's job is not viewed as harshly as it once was. The loss of a job is much more common in today's changing work

*Part I* Career Planning and Development in Nursing

environment. Three key ways of losing a job are through restructuring and layoffs, being fired, and being asked to take early retirement or voluntary separation (Helfand, 1999).

Although nurses often have plans related to returning to school, most do not have a plan if they were to lose their job. If you do not have a "what if I should lose my job tomorrow" plan, you should begin to develop one. To do this you need to first ask yourself the question, "What is the worst thing that could happen?" By being proactive, you can anticipate possible scenarios and develop a plan for dealing with each of them. This will help you realize that you do have choices, even when it may very well feel as if you have none.

Once you have heard that you are losing your job, you may experience the five emotions associated with grieving. Helfand (1999) describes how it is common to experience emotions of denial, anger, bargaining, depression and, lastly, acceptance. Two other emotions that many experience are fear and shame. Fear often occurs between denial and anger and is related to family concerns such as how bills will be paid and whether you will ever work again. Shame may occur after anger and before depression. Do not be surprised if you also experience feelings such as disbelief, disappointment, despair, hurt, sadness, betrayal, self-pity and, sometimes, relief. Although you may experience some, many, or only a few of these emotions, it is important to have support systems in place that can support you through this difficult time. You will need those that are sympathetic as you go through the grieving process, but you will also need others who will challenge you to move forward to find something better.

You also need to create a routine and get organized about your job search and life. To keep you organized, it is helpful to create daily schedules of things to do. Keep records of who you contact, and make sure to schedule time for yourself.

Soon after you have learned that you have lost your job, you need to begin exploring the support systems provided by the organization and the external community. Governments usually have documents that outline what your employer must provide. You also may be eligible to participate in government programs that provide practical support and information. Many organizations provide severance packages; however, they often do not make them public, and so it will be important for you to ask about them. Severance benefits can include items such as severance pay, employee assistance programs, outplacement counselling, and payment for unused vacation time. If you feel you have been treated unfairly, you can always consult your union or a lawyer.

Many who lose their job experience fear related to financial concerns. When you have lost your job, it is important to review your financial situation and identify information such as that listed in the box on p. 61.

Once you have the information, you need to sit down with pen and paper and itemize all your expenses and revenue sources, both current and potential. This information will assist you in developing a financial plan to support you until you find new employment.

| *Financial Assessment* |
| --- |
| • How much money do I need to live each month?<br>• How much money do I owe?<br>• Do I have an emergency or contingency fund?<br>• Do I have friends or family who could help? |

While you look for a new job, it is important to take care of yourself. During difficult times, many try to either eat or starve away their problems and get little exercise. It is important to eat a well-balanced diet and to exercise to be mentally alert, increase your energy level, and help you deal most effectively with the stress. You may find it helpful to join a health club, participate in some method of relaxation, take a trip, and do some self-reflection as you plan your next step. Seeking professional help during this difficult time may also be useful. This is not a sign of weakness; it is a sign of strength. No one wants this to happen. By being proactive and creating a plan for what to do if you lose your job, you will be prepared. You will be taking control of your career. The good news is that many people often end up with much better jobs than the ones they left!

## CONCLUSION

A strategic career plan is a comprehensive way to assist you in reaching your career vision. With a well-developed career plan, you will be able to define your short-term and long-term goals and the action steps needed to achieve your goals. Your career plan will enable you to be proactive. It will assist you in taking risks and facing your internal and external barriers. You will also be able to recognize and take advantage of career opportunities when they occur.

Your career plan belongs to you. You have created it based on your dreams. As your dreams change, so will your plan. It is an ongoing work in progress. Throughout your career life span, you will continually modify it as new opportunities and growth are achieved. With a well-developed career plan, you will be well on your way to taking control of your future.

## REFERENCES

Alberta Advanced Education and Career Development. (1999). *Multiple choices: Planning your career for the 21st century.* Edmonton, Alberta, Canada: Author.

Foord Kirk, J. (1996). *Survivability: Career strategies for the new world of work.* Kelowna, British Columbia, Canada: Kirkfoord Communications.

Helfand, D.P. (1999). Career change: Everything you need to know to meet new challenges and take control of your career (2nd ed.). Chicago: VGM Career Horizons.

Kaye, B. (1993). *Up is not the only way: A guide to developing workforce talent.* Washington, DC: Career Systems.

Sher, B. (1983). *Wishcraft: How to get what you really want.* New York: Ballantine Books.

Simonsen, P. (2000). *Career compass: Navigating your career strategically in the new century.* Palo, Alto, CA: Davies-Black:

Von Oech, R. (1986). *A kick in the seat of the pants.* New York: Harper & Row.

White, S.K. (1990). Reach for the sky. *Heart & Lung, 19*(3), 28A-39A.

## FURTHER READING

Career Development (2002). *Beliefs and Assumptions.* Retrieved October 19, 2002 http://careerplanning.about.com/gi/dynamic/offsite.htm?site=http: www.nwc. edu/career/planning/phase/workvalues.htm.

Feather, F. (1996). *Canada's best careers guide* (3rd ed.). Toronto, Canada: Warwick.

Jeffers, S. (1987). *Feel the fear and do it anyway.* New York: Fawcett Columbine.

Kanchier, C. (2000). *Dare to change your job and your life.* Indianapolis: JIST Works.

Siber, L. (1999). *Career management for the creative person.* New York: Three Rivers Press.

Yancer, D., & Klausen, J. (1997). *Navigate your career transition: Strategies for nurse leaders.* Chicago: American Hospital Publishing Inc.

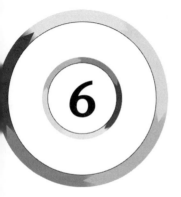

# Marketing Yourself

Sue Bookey-Bassett, RN, BScN, MEd

**Sue Bookey-Bassett** is a professional development consultant in nursing. She was formerly a program manager at the Registered Nurses Association of Ontario's (RNAO) Centre for Professional Nursing Excellence, where her work included providing individual career counselling, workshops and seminars.

## Author Reflections

*I believe that a customized self-marketing plan has been key in finding work that fits with my interests and skills. Résumés have opened doors and interviews have given me the opportunity to really demonstrate my skills and talents. I have personally seen the benefits of building networks that have contributed to achieving my professional goals.*

*Whatever you do or dream you can do—begin it. Boldness has genius and power and magic in it.*

*Goethe*

In the previous chapters you learned about the changing world of health care and its impact on nurses' work. You also read about the importance of doing a comprehensive self-assessment and reality check. Now that you have completed your strategic career plan, you are ready to begin looking for career opportunities that are meaningful and satisfying to you. The purpose of this chapter is to provide you with information and tools to help you develop an effective self-marketing strategy that you can use to take control of your career and your future. This chapter begins with a discussion about marketing yourself and why doing so is crucial for nurses in their search for a rewarding career. Various strategies are presented, including specific examples for marketing yourself on paper (e.g., résumé and business cards) and in person (networking and interviewing).

## WHAT IS MARKETING, WHY IS IT IMPORTANT, AND HOW DO WE DO IT?

Searching for work in the 21st century is not simply about sending résumés and answering classified ads for positions in which you are interested. It is a much more dynamic process that includes marketing or selling yourself as a product and as a package of knowledge and accomplishments, not just past titles and job history (Enelow, 2002; McGowan, 2002). In other words, you must convince potential employers why they should hire or appoint you and what you have to offer them.

In completing your self-assessment, you will have identified your values and beliefs, past experiences, accomplishments, strengths, and areas for improvement. You can use these facts to determine how you want to present or market yourself to others to meet your career goals. As you learned in Chapter 2, the current health care environment is complex and volatile and thus has many opportunities for career growth, but it also has many challenges. Now that you have a vision and a plan, you need a specific set of strategies that position you to get what you want. Self-marketing is about how you present yourself to others. It includes making yourself visible, establishing a network, finding a mentor, and enhancing your written and verbal communication skills. Developing a strategy for self-marketing can assist you in moving from the planning phase to the results phase in achieving your career goals. When marketing yourself, you are in control of how and to whom you want to present yourself and what it is you want people to know about you.

## Marketing Strategies

Throughout daily interactions with patients, peers, and other professionals, nurses have many opportunities to present themselves to—and to influence—others. As we do this, we create a certain image and send a particular message about who we are. In fact, you are your own best marketer. It is how you look, comport yourself, dress, and behave that makes the earliest impression and is the first step in self-marketing. This presentation of self is not about trying to be someone else but rather about ensuring that you present the person you are in the best possible light. Before you begin to use all the other marketing tools and strategies available, consider the "product" that is you. What type of direct and indirect feedback do you get when you present yourself and your ideas to clients, friends, and colleagues? The notion of marketing ourselves is often uncomfortable because we think it means manipulating or deceiving others—but it is exactly the opposite. It is having the confidence in who we are and in what we want to do and projecting that to others. That is the first step. After we understand and deal with our self-image, we can go on to make use of the other marketing tools and strategies.

### Networking

Establishing a network is one of the most powerful strategies to achieve your career goals, not only for a specific job search but for lifelong career management (Enelow, 2002). Networking is key to keeping informed about what is happening in nursing and in health care and of how the emerging trends and issues impact nurses' work so you can position yourself strategically and maintain your professional visibility. It is about building relationships with others to meet career goals. It is a mutual process that may involve the exchange of information and resources both in person and in writing. Networking is not about asking other people for jobs but rather about asking others to help you meet your career goals. This may be accomplished through gathering more information, asking for referrals to others, or seeking new opportunities.

The process of developing a network begins by thinking of people who share your values and interests and who may be helpful to you—peers, nurse managers, clinical resources, human resources staff, and other professionals. Think of nurses who are doing the type of work that you would like to do, and arrange to meet with them. Other potential people to include in your network are university or college nursing professors, previous employers, preceptors, and nursing leaders within health care organizations and professional associations, as well as family and friends. Once you have made a list of people to include in your network, contact them; be specific about what you are looking for and what you would like them to do for you. Also remember who you are and what you can do for them. Who you know is not as important as who knows you. People need to know who you are in order to help you.

Building your network is an ongoing process, and people in your network will change over time. Continue to develop your network by participating in committees and projects and by attending workshops or conferences. Formal education and involvement in professional organizations can also help expand your professional network. Take the opportunity to meet and speak with others. You never know where new relationships may lead.

### Support Groups

A support group is a group of people on whom you can count for both personal and professional support. The group may include people in your network along with others who are interested in supporting you as you work to achieve your career goals. Select people who are positive and will contribute to your confidence in working toward your goals. Of course, select individuals whom you want to support and help as well. Use your support group for honest feedback and emotional support when you need extra encouragement, such as when you are about to take a risk.

### Finding a Mentor

Acquiring a mentor can provide the additional support and guidance necessary to help you transform your career dreams into reality. A mentor is someone who is interested in you and your career and is willing and able to help you meet specific career goals (Bower, 2000; Case, 1997). In nursing, mentors are often more experienced nurses who know the ins and outs of the health care environment, have good connections, and have more access to information than younger, less experienced nurses. Nursing mentors have often contributed to the nursing world in a specific way and are interested in sharing their knowledge and fostering leadership skills in less experienced nurses. Depending on what specific help you are looking for, you may decide that a non-nurse may be a better choice for a mentor. A mentor can support you in scanning your environment, conducting your self-assessment, and developing a specific career plan. Mentors may be able to open doors to enhance your professional visibility and success by helping you learn ways to become more politically savvy and to meet the right people.

Mentorship can take many forms and can facilitate your personal and professional development. Some mentor relationships are formal, whereas others are informal (Bower, 2000). A true mentor relationship is one that mutually benefits both the mentor and the learner (protégé). It is often a long-term relationship that is chosen, not assigned. It conveys a mutual respect, a common interest, and a desire to grow professionally.

When choosing a mentor, look for someone who is watching you grow professionally and who has the following characteristics: patience, enthusiasm, knowledge, a sense of humour, and respect (Fawcett, 2002). Also consider the mentor's (1) leadership style; (2) time and willingness to devote to you as the protégé; (3) skills to advise, teach, counsel, and refer; and (4) availability to support you in achieving your goals (Bower, 2000). Get to know a potential mentor by volunteering to work on similar projects or by choosing to sit on a committee of which he or she is a member. If your mentor does not work in the same organization, find ways to meet with him or her to discuss your goals. It is important to determine whether there is a good fit between you and your potential mentor. Both parties need to commit to the relationship. Remember to discuss what you have to offer and what you are seeking from the mentoring relationship. You need to know what you want in order to ask for it.

You may feel uncomfortable about approaching a potential mentor. However, keep in mind that mentors can also benefit from the relationship with a protégé. It gives them an opportunity to contribute to their profession and/or society by developing others and helping them expand their networks.

## Marketing Yourself on Paper

### *Résumés*

A well-constructed résumé is an important part of self-marketing. An effective résumé represents your knowledge, skills, and achievements in such a convincing way that the reader can get an immediate sense of who you are and what you can do for them. A résumé creates a first impression, and its main purpose is to get you an interview or an opportunity to present yourself in person.

Creating a résumé requires time, patience, and practice. There is no such thing as a generic or one-size-fits-all résumé. To be most effective, your résumé must be customized for each and every opportunity you pursue (Enelow, 2002; Hacker, 1999). It should include components of your self-assessment (i.e., your knowledge, skills, and specific and measurable achievements). A résumé should not just restate a job description. Today's employers are looking for what and how results were achieved. Therefore when describing your achievements, be sure to quantify them if possible (Kursmark, 2001).

Before customizing a résumé, you need to know something about the position for which you are applying. What qualifications is the employer looking for and how do your knowledge, skills, and accomplishments relate to the position? It is also helpful to know something about the organization (i.e., What are the organization's values related to patient care? Does your résumé reflect similar values?). To assist you in customizing your résumé, consider using a format that reflects your personal style and career goals but allows for customization of specific sections as necessary. Sending the same résumé to many potential employers is easy but can be inefficient and discouraging; all you are likely to get is a number of rejection letters. Customizing takes more time and effort but in the long run will yield more satisfying results (Hacker, 1999).

*What is the Difference Between a Résumé and Curriculum Vitae (CV)?* The terms *résumé* and *curriculum vitae (CV)* are often used interchangeably, but they are actually two different documents. A résumé is a summary document, usually two to three pages, that highlights your education, professional background, and accomplishments. Figure 6-1 is an outline for a CV. It is a detailed and all-encompassing document that describes your professional and academic interests and reflects your entire career to date. A CV is usually used to apply for grants, scholarships, awards, and academic appointments. A résumé, on the other hand, is most often used to apply for a specific job or position. If you are unsure as to which document an employer requires, you can always call to clarify.

*Types of Résumés*

CHRONOLOGICAL STYLE. In general, there are two basic résumé styles: chronological and functional. Some people prefer to combine the two styles into what is often referred to as a hybrid style.

The chronological format is the most common and more traditional type of nursing résumé. In a chronological résumé, work history and education are described in reverse chronological order, with the most recent experiences appearing first. Chronological résumés emphasize dates, position titles, responsibilities, and the names and locations of previous employers (Kursmark, 2001). This style is most often used to demonstrate career progression by showing positions of increased responsibility or preparation. See Figure 6-2 for a sample of a chronological résumé.

1. **Name, Address, Phone, Fax, E-mail.**

2. **Education:** Degrees, certificates and diplomas granted, name and location of institution.

3. **Academic Honours and Awards:** Name of award, name of agency granting award.

4. **Professional/Community Honours and Awards:** May be combined with Item 3.

5. **Current Position:** Position title, employing agency. If an academic position, follow this section with sections on undergraduate courses taught, graduate courses taught, and Masters or PhD students supervised.

6. **Previous Positions:** Position title, employing agency, brief description of the role.

7. **Funded Research:** Grant name, granting agency, amount of grant.

8. **Publications:** Use a consistent and recognizable format to list your publications, such as the APA style. Use the following subsections: peer-reviewed, chapters in books, book reviews, and other publications.

9. **Academic Presentations:** Include peer-reviewed abstracts or papers.

10. **Professional/Community Presentations:** Include speeches and non-refereed papers.

11. **Peer Review Activities:** Grant reviews, journal reviews.

12. **University/Academic Boards and Committees:** Can be divided into university-wide and faculty or department categories.

13. **Professional Consultations:** Work you may have done for organizations, professional associations, and other organizations.

14. **Professional Boards and Committees.**

15. **Community Service.**

16. **Special Appointments:** Any government or other appointments that you want to highlight separately.

Figure **6-1.** Outline for a curriculum vitae (CV).

## Susan Jones, RN, BScN
Street Address
Any City, Province K2S 4M4
Phone Number
E-mail address

**Career Objective:**
To obtain an RN position in a maternal-newborn program in a teaching hospital environment that will allow me to utilize my X years of maternal-newborn experience and provide high-quality nursing care to childbearing families.

## EDUCATION

2002     **Bachelor of Science in Nursing**
         Name of University
         City, Province

2002     **Breastfeeding Certificate**
         Name of Institution
         City, Province

1997     **Registered Nurse Diploma**
         Name of College
         City, Province

## HONOURS AND AWARDS

2001     Most Valuable Nurse, Maternal-Newborn Services
         General Hospital
         City, Province

## EMPLOYMENT HISTORY

1998 to present     **Staff Nurse, Combined Care, Maternal-Newborn Program**
                    Community Hospital, City, Province
                    Provided comprehensive nursing care to new families, including patient assessment, teaching, discharge planning, and referral to community resources.

                    Accomplishments: Preceptor to new staff nurses; clinical resource nurse for unit; member of the patient education committee; taught prenatal classes; developed  dads only  prenatal class.

Figure **6-2.** Sample of a chronological résumé.                    *Continued*

| 1997 to 1998 | **Staff Nurse, General Medical Unit, Adult Medicine Program**<br>Community Hospital, City, Province<br>Provided total nursing care to patients with a variety of medical diagnoses, including diabetes and cardiac, renal, and pulmonary disease. Coordinated care in collaboration with members of the multidisciplinary team.<br><br>Accomplishments: Assisted in development of a patient/family education centre on the unit; member of patient education committee. |
|---|---|

## COMMITTEE PARTICIPATION

| 1997 to present | Member, Patient Education Committee<br>Community Hospital |
|---|---|

## PROFESSIONAL MEMBERSHIPS

| 1997 to present | Provincial Nurses Association |
|---|---|
| 1997 to present | Canadian Nurses Association |
| 1997 to present | Association of Women s Health, Obstetrical and Neonatal Nurses |

## PUBLICATIONS

Jones, S. (2000). What new parents need to know. *Name of Journal, volume,* pages.

## CONTINUING EDUCATION/PROFESSIONAL DEVELOPMENT

| 2001 | Provincial Nursing Association Annual General Meeting<br>City, Province |
|---|---|
| 1998 | National Perinatal Nursing Conference<br>City, Province |

## COMMUNITY PARTICIPATION

| 2000 to present | Guest speaker to new parent groups |
|---|---|

Figure **6-2,** cont'd For legend, see p. 69.

FUNCTIONAL STYLE. The functional résumé highlights an individual's skills and accomplishments using various categories. This style allows the opportunity to accentuate transferable skills and puts less emphasis on the previous jobs held or on academic preparation. A functional résumé may be more relevant if you are changing roles (i.e., moving from a staff nurse position to an educator or management role). It can also be used for those nurses who may be seeking employment in non-traditional nursing roles or outside of the health care sector. The functional résumé allows you to highlight your skills related to the qualifications the employer is looking for. Figure 6-3 shows a sample of a functional résumé.

---

**Susan Jones, RN, BScN**
Street Address
City, Province, Postal Code
Phone Number
E-mail address

**Career Objective:**
To obtain an RN position in a maternal-newborn program in a teaching hospital environment that will allow me to utilize my X years of maternal-newborn experience and provide high-quality nursing care to childbearing families.

**ACHIEVEMENTS**

**Clinical Expertise**

X years of clinical nursing with post-partum patients and their families. Clinical resource nurse for peers on the unit. Competent in providing all aspects of nursing care. Completed breastfeeding certificate.

**Leadership**

Member of patient education committee and preceptor for new staff members. Assisted in development of a patient/family education centre on medical unit.

**Education**

Revised patient education materials for unit. Co-taught prenatal classes to expectant families with emphasis on *Breastfeeding Your Newborn*. Developed special *Dads Only Class*.

---

Figure **6-3.** Sample of a functional résumé.                          *Continued*

## WORK EXPERIENCE

1998 to present     **Staff Nurse, Combined Care, Maternal-Newborn Program**
Community Hospital, City, Province

1997 to 1998     **Staff Nurse, General Medical Unit, Adult Medicine Program**
Community Hospital, City, Province

## EDUCATION

2002     Bachelor of Science in Nursing
Name of University
City, Province

2002     Breastfeeding Certificate
Name of Institution
City, Province

1997     Registered Nurse Diploma
Name of College
City, Province

## HONOURS AND AWARDS

2001     Most Valuable Nurse, Maternal-Newborn Services
General Hospital
City, Province

## COMMITTEE PARTICIPATION

1997 to present     Member, Patient Education Committee
Community Hospital

## PROFESSIONAL MEMBERSHIPS

1997 to present     Provincial Nurses Association
1997 to present     Canadian Nurses Association
1997 to present     Association of Women's Health, Obstetrical and Neonatal Nurses

## PUBLICATIONS

Jones, S. (2000). What new parents need to know. *Name of Journal,* volume, pages.

Figure **6-3,** cont'd For legend, see p. 71.

---

**CONTINUING EDUCATION/PROFESSIONAL DEVELOPMENT**

| 2001 | Provincial Nursing Association Annual General Meeting<br>City, Province |
|------|------------------------------------------------------------------------|
| 1998 | National Perinatal Nursing Conference<br>City, Province |

**COMMUNITY PARTICIPATION**

| 2000 to present | Guest speaker to new parent groups |
|-----------------|------------------------------------|

Figure **6-3,** cont'd For legend, see p. 71.

HYBRID STYLE. The hybrid résumé combines the strengths of the chronological and functional résumés. It emphasizes career continuity as in the chronological style, but it also highlights the themes of expertise and accomplishments as reflected in the functional style. Figure 6-4 illustrates an example of a hybrid résumé.

### Creating Your Résumé

Creating a résumé can be a very intimidating experience. It requires time and effort. Ideally résumés should be kept up-to-date on an ongoing basis; however, most people tend not to look at their résumé unless they are planning a change in employment or have experienced a job loss. Before you begin, take some time to reflect on your self-assessment and on your career plan. Rushing to prepare a résumé without having a clear picture in your mind of the message you want to give will make the task much more difficult and the outcome less useful.

The next section describes what information to include under each of the potential headings in your résumé. Remember that these are guidelines; you can tailor specific sections to meet your individual needs or the needs of the particular employer. As you design your résumé, think about how you want to market your skills and abilities to the employer. What do you have to offer?

*Career Objective or a Career Summary.* A career objective is a statement of what you are looking for (i.e., type of work or position). Be as specific as possible so that employers will know what you are interested in. For example, if you are interested in obstetrical nursing, state that rather than the generic line "a position as a RN." Being specific ensures that the right person (i.e., the person doing the hiring) will read it.

A career summary is used by experienced nurses to create a strong positive impression by summarizing strengths, accomplishments, expertise, and career interests. The advantage of the career summary is that it whets the appetite of prospective employers and encourages them to read on for more details.

# Rob Smith, RN, BScN
Street Address
City, Province, Postal Code
Phone Number
E-mail address

**Objective:** To obtain a nursing management position in a geriatric extended-care facility, including staff development, education, and supervision of nursing staff and other direct care providers.

## SUMMARY OF QUALIFICATIONS

- Clinical expertise and experience in all aspects of geriatric care
- Acting nurse manager for 6 months
- Demonstrated skill in teaching and supervising registered and non-registered care providers
- Committed to excellence in nursing practice and challenging others to strive for excellence

## RELEVANT EXPERIENCE

### LEADERSHIP

- Coordinated and supervised health care team members responsible for 24-hour care of geriatric patients at Eastside Nursing Home, Unit A
- Initiated unit implementation of Best Practice Guidelines related to pressure ulcers
- Managed revision of existing patient care policies, including patient restraint and family visitation to enhance patient safety and satisfaction
- Decreased staff absenteeism by introducing self-scheduling for nursing staff

### Staff Development

- Met with all nursing staff to develop individual learning goals for the next year
- Clinical resource nurse for peers prior to acting manager role
- Preceptor to new nursing staff for the past 4 years
- Worked with corporate organizational development team to provide 2-day workshops for staff on client-centred care

### Clinical Excellence

- 10 years progressive nursing experience in geriatric settings
- National Nurses Association Certification in Gerontological Nursing (2000)
- 3 years part-time nursing faculty for Name of Community College teaching gerontological nursing as part of post-RN programs
- Nominated by peers for Professional Association's Nursing Practice Award (2001)

Figure **6-4.** Sample of a hybrid résumé.

## WORK EXPERIENCE

June 2002 to
December 2002

**Acting Nursing Manager**
Eastside Nursing Home, City, Province
Responsible for all aspects of patient care on Unit
  A, including management of human and fiscal
  resources, care delivery, quality management,
  staff and patient education

1999 to present

**Part-Time Faculty Post-RN Continuing
Education Program**
College, City, Province
Prepared course outline and selected readings list;
  delivered lectures and arranged for guest
  speakers; wrote and graded exams; advised
  students on clinical and academic issues

1992 to
June 2002

**Staff Nurse, Unit A**
Employer, City, Province
Responsible for providing all aspects of patient
  care, including supervision of non-registered
  staff and nursing students. Developed
  collaborative relationships with other
  members of the health care team and
  family members to ensure the highest
  quality of patient care

## EDUCATION

1999 to present

Master of Nursing (in progress)
University, City, Province

1994

Certificate in Gerontological Nursing
College, City, Province

1992

Bachelor of Science in Nursing
University, City, Province

## PUBLICATIONS

Smith, R. (2000). Pursuing excellence in clinical practice through
certification. *Journal.* Vol., pages.

Figure **6-4,** cont'd For legend, see p. 74.

---

### COMMITTEE PARTICIPATION

| | |
|---|---|
| 2002 | Nursing Practice Committee, Accreditation Team |
| 2001 | Healthy Work Environment Task Force |
| 1999 | Staff Development Committee |

### PRESENTATIONS

Smith, R. (date). Name of presentation. Name of conference. City, Province.

### PROFESSIONAL MEMBERSHIPS

| | |
|---|---|
| 2000 to present | Gerontological Nurses Association |
| 1994 to present | Provincial Professional Nurses Association |

### COMMUNITY ACTIVITIES

| | |
|---|---|
| 2000 to present | Guest speaker for Healthy Heart Program for Seniors |

---

Figure **6-4,** cont'd For legend, see p. 74.

*Education.* Education can be separated into two sections: (1) education that yields a diploma, degree, or certificate, and (2) other continuing education. Your continuing education should appear in a separate section later in your résumé (after your work experience), and it is best labeled "Professional Development." As your career progresses, this section can become quite lengthy; therefore include only professional development activities relevant to the position for which you are applying, and label this section "Selected Professional Development Activities."

*Honours and Awards.* If you have received honours or awards from your workplace, academic institution, or professional nursing association, highlight them in a separate category to accentuate their merit. Remember to include the year the award was presented and the name of the sponsoring organization.

*Work Experience.* Many different terms are used to describe this section: *employment history, professional accomplishments, work history, employment experience,* and *professional experience.* Choose the term you prefer, and remember that the information in this section should reflect your career progression by describing your ongoing contributions and accomplishments. An accomplishment refers to those activities in which you went beyond what you were hired to do. They are not items on a job description. They are situations in which you identified a challenge, used a specific approach, and achieved a successful outcome. Accomplishments represent times when you achieved a personal or professional best. How did your accomplishments make a difference in your workplace? Try to be specific and include measurable results of your accomplishments. This will help you differentiate yourself as an achiever.

In a functional résumé, there is less detail regarding your past jobs and more emphasis on your major skills and accomplishments. In general, people choose two to four functional headings that are customized to match a specific position. For example, if a specific position requires skills such as leadership, communication, clinical expertise, and research, you can design your résumé to include these skills as your functional headings. Using key words or sector-specific jargon can be an effective marketing strategy (Enelow, 2001).

*Professional Memberships and Affiliations.* In this section, list current and relevant memberships and affiliations. Include any offices or leadership positions you have held. Involvement in professional organizations demonstrates that you are keeping up-to-date with professional issues.

*Publications and Presentations.* Publications and presentations demonstrate your expertise and knowledge in a particular area, as well as your ability to engage in research and scholarly writing. Include written materials you have authored and co-authored, including patient education materials, professional articles, or teaching tools. If you have numerous publications, provide the most recent and relevant ones (the past 7 years is considered appropriate). As a co-author or a member of a research team, you are entitled to be cited as a contributor on any publication. Make sure to negotiate this when you are recruited for such projects.

*Community/Volunteer Experience.* Most of us are involved in our communities, either professionally or personally. Include experiences (along with dates and names of organizations) that are relevant to the type of work you are seeking. It is useful to include volunteer experience that has provided you with skills you may not have developed in your paid work. This section should serve as a means of enhancing the breadth of your accomplishments.

*References.* It is not desirable to include the names of references on your résumé, although they are commonly included. Just like everything else in your résumé, you want your references to be relevant to the position and the organization. If the employer requires references before the interview, you can include them on a separate piece of paper. Some people include the line "references available on request" at the end of the résumé. However, because it is assumed you will provide such references when asked to do so, it is a redundant line.

*Other Tips.* For more tips on creating résumés, see Figure 6-5.

### Using Technology: Electronic Résumés

Technology has had a huge impact on the job search process, and health care and nursing have not been excluded. Having an electronic résumé is another important self-marketing tool. In fact, many hiring managers and recruiters prefer to receive résumés by e-mail (Whitcomb & Kendall, 2002).

What exactly is an electronic résumé? E-résumés come in various formats, such as a MS Word attachment, a text version, a PDF file, a résumé posted to

| Résumé Do's | Résumé Don'ts |
|---|---|
| • Print on good quality paper using a laser printer.<br>• Use preferred colours of paper: white, ivory, or pale gray.<br>• Font size should be 10 or 12 point.<br>• Font type should be easy to read (e.g., Arial or Times New Roman).<br>• Send cover letter on matching paper.<br>• Length should be 2 to 3 pages.<br>• Emphasize accomplishments and results.<br>• If faxing a résumé, always send a hard copy.<br>• Customize your résumé for each position to which you apply. | • Do not enclose a photograph.<br>• Do not include birth date, nationality, or religious or political affiliations.<br>• Do not mention salary.<br>• Do not repeat your job description.<br>• Do not send a résumé without a cover letter.<br>• Do not send a résumé on your current employer's letterhead.<br>• Do not attach reference letters to your résumé.<br>• Do not send out résumés indiscriminately. |

Figure **6-5.** Résumé do's and don'ts.

a job board, a Web résumé/portfolio, or a CD-ROM résumé/portfolio (Dixson, 2001). To e-mail a résumé successfully, the file must be in the proper electronic format. Be sure to check with employers regarding which format they require. Although technology may enhance the timelines with which individuals can apply for positions, it also poses risks such as attached viruses and corrupt files.

Various electronic formats and tips for electronic résumés are highlighted in the boxes on p. 79 (Dixson, 2001).

Having a basic e-résumé is an essential tool for nurses searching for new career opportunities. For further resources to create your e-résumé, refer to books on electronic résumés, career centres, and your professional associations.

### An Essential Component: The Cover Letter

A résumé must always be accompanied by a one-page cover letter. The purpose of a cover letter is to encourage prospective employers to read your résumé in more detail in order to determine how your experience and abilities can benefit their organization. The cover letter should be written after your résumé but should not be a repetition of the résumé itself.

A cover letter has three main components. The first component is an opening statement describing the position you are applying for, how you learned about the opportunity, and how your specific skills and abilities match the

### Formatting Electronic Résumés

- **MS Word Files:** Sent as attachments; easy to send but can be edited at the recipient's end.
- **Text only (ASCII):** Compatible with all systems; fully formatted résumé is saved as text; paste the text résumé into the body of your message preceded by a brief cover letter.
- **PDF file:** Preserves the intended format; need Adobe Acrobat reader software to open.
- **Posted résumés:** Posting your résumé to a job board, company, or recruiter website; often requires using an online résumé builder or a predefined template; can be quick and efficient but may not allow for customization; all applicants must use the same template to apply. Nursing and health care employers have been using posted résumés for several years.
- **Web résumé:** A formatted HTML version of a résumé on the World Wide Web; allows for unique and individual customization using colour and design; your résumé has its own website and can be viewed by anyone at any time.
- **Web career portfolios:** A creative way to market your skills and knowledge by constructing a URL; provides visual evidence as to your wide range of skills and abilities.
- **CD-ROM résumés/career portfolios:** More prevalent in other sectors; can incorporate the use of multimedia technology; come in business card size, which can be an impressive way to distribute résumés at career fairs or employer open houses.

### Electronic Résumé Tips

- Check with employer regarding the preferred format.
- Be familiar with the advantages and disadvantages of each format.
- Use key words when constructing your résumé. Key words are "words associated with a specific industry, profession or job function, that clearly and succinctly communicate a specific message" (Dixson, 2001). To find key words, review job postings, corporate websites, classified ads, and job descriptions. Key words should be used when customizing your résumé for specific positions.

employer's requirements. You want this statement to quickly capture the reader's attention. The second component is the main body of the letter and should emphasize why you are interested in the position and what you have to offer. Mention that your enclosed résumé provides more details regarding your qualifications. Remember, the goal of the cover letter is to convince prospective employers that they will benefit if they decide to find out how you can meet their needs. The last component is the closing paragraph, in which you request an interview to discuss the possible fit between what the employer is looking for and what you have to offer (Davis, 2001). In today's competitive and rapidly changing world of work, nurses must use clear goals and creative strategies when designing cover letters.

Figure 6-6 provides a list of what a cover letter must contain. Figure 6-7 illustrates a sample cover letter.

### Business Cards

Another self-marketing strategy to consider is a personal business card. You may already have business cards related to your current position, but these will not be appropriate if you are in the process of looking for alternative opportunities. Having a personal business card when you are networking with others is more impressive than fumbling with pen and paper.

Your business card represents who you are, so you want it to be attractive and look professional. It should include your name, credentials, address, telephone, fax, and e-mail addresses. You can create your business cards on your home computer, or they can be purchased through a print shop quickly and inexpensively. You may want to see examples of the business cards of your friends and colleagues before ordering your own cards. Business cards are great tools for networking at job fairs, conferences, or other professional meetings.

### Writing for Publication

Writing about your work as a nurse offers further opportunities to market your knowledge and skills. There are a variety of media in which to publish your work. Your first publication does not need to be in a scholarly, peer-reviewed nursing journal. It could be in the newsletters of your workplace or professional association, in clinical journals, or in letters to the editor of local and national newspapers.

What can you write about? Nurses can write about various aspects of their work, such as new methods of delivering patient care, patient outcomes as a result of nursing care, career satisfaction, how to demonstrate leadership, and how to influence others. Write about what you know: how nurses make a difference in patient care. Writing also demonstrates your knowledge

---

A cover letter must:
- Be targeted to each specific employer
- Be addressed to the person most likely making the hiring decision
- Convey personal warmth and enthusiasm
- Be proofread and proofread again to check for spelling or grammatical errors

Figure **6-6.** Cover letter musts.

Street Address
City, Province
Postal Code
Phone Number

Date

Ms. Jane Smith
Program Director
Palliative Care Program
General Health Centre
City, Province, Postal Code

Dear Ms. Smith:

I am writing in response to the advertisement posted on the General Health Centre's website for a staff nurse position in the expanded Palliative Care Program.

As a staff nurse working in an oncology unit for 5 years, I am excited about the expansion of your palliative care program and the opportunities it will create for patients and staff. Through my experience to date, I have developed clinical expertise and in-depth knowledge in caring for oncology patients. I have also participated in several initiatives with community agencies to facilitate early discharge, which has increased my awareness of the need to expand the palliative care program at your facility. My enclosed résumé provides further details about my qualifications, skills, and accomplishments.

I would appreciate the opportunity to discuss my potential contribution to your organization's palliative care program. I look forward to hearing from you. Thank you for your consideration.

Sincerely,

(Your signature)

Katherine Black, RN, BScN

Enclosure: Résumé

Figure **6-7.** Sample cover letter.

regarding a specific nursing or health care issue. Be sure to include your contact information on any publications so that others can contact you for more information. Any chance to present your knowledge and abilities in writing creates further opportunities for self-marketing.

## Marketing Yourself in Person

The previous sections discussed strategies for marketing yourself on paper. This section describes some of the strategies for marketing yourself in person, including interviewing, making presentations, and acting as a mentor. With all of these strategies, it is important to keep in mind that you, and how you feel about and present yourself, are critical in self-marketing.

### The Interview: An Excellent Marketing Opportunity

You have just received a call from one of your employers of choice. It's true; they want you to appear for an interview in one week. What do you need to do to prepare yourself for this marketing opportunity?

In today's world of work, the interview is a crucial step in landing a new job. In all fields of work, the interviewing process has become more complex. Nurses may be faced with various types of interviews and need to be prepared to sell themselves and their skills in a variety of ways. Developing strong interview skills is essential for career success.

The interview is the most important component of the job search process. Getting an interview is a sign that the employer thinks you have the qualifications for the job. It is up to you to sell yourself to the potential employer by presenting yourself as the best candidate for the job. It is an opportunity to convince the employer that there is a strong fit between your skills and knowledge and those required by the position. You must clearly articulate what skills you have to offer and how you have demonstrated those skills through past experience. The box below lists some of the interview methods being used by employers.

### Types of Interviews

- Single interviewer
- Group or panel interview
- Behavioural interview
- Serial interview
- Telephone interview

*Preparing for an Interview: An Essential Step for Success.* Contrary to some beliefs, interviewing is a serious process. We can no longer "wing it." To be successful in interviews, preparation is essential. The box on p. 83 lists some general guidelines to help you prepare for an interview.

Investing time and effort in preparing for an interview can result in a successful interview and, ultimately, a job offer. Many resources are available to

---

### Preparing for the Interview

1. Find out what type of interview to expect. How many people will be interviewing you? Who is the contact person?
2. Confirm the date, time, and location of the interview, particularly if an organization has more than one site. On the day of the interview, be sure you know how to get to the interview site, and allow extra time to get there.
3. Do some research about the organization. What are their values, mission, and philosophy? What is the strategic plan? Is the organization downsizing, merging, or expanding programs? Have there been any recent staff layoffs? Much of this information can be found on employer websites.
4. Review the ad or job description of the position for which you are being interviewed. Be able to articulate how your skills, expertise, and accomplishments meet the position requirements.
5. Anticipate potential questions you may be asked during the interview, and prepare answers to those questions.
6. Practice interviewing with a friend, colleague, mentor, instructor, or career coach. Ask for feedback on how you answered the questions. This can be a very helpful strategy if done in a serious but non-threatening manner.
7. Bring extra copies of your résumé to the interview.
8. Be polite and respectful to everyone in the organization. Receptionists may play an informal role in the hiring process.
9. Prepare some questions to ask the interviewer(s). Include questions that will allow you to learn more about the organization and the position itself.

---

help you prepare for an interview. Some resources include books related to career planning and interviewing; friends, colleagues, and people in your support group and network; career coaches in career centres; and professional associations. Choose resources based on your specific needs and learning style.

*The Actual Interview.* The day has come, and it is now time to go to the interview. Plan to arrive 10 to 15 minutes before the interview is scheduled to begin. While waiting for your interview, use the time to review the job description, your résumé, and your questions. If you are nervous, try doing some deep-breathing exercises to relax.

PRESENTING YOURSELF. Remember that an interview is an excellent self-marketing opportunity and is your first chance to make a good impression. Dress in a professional and conservative manner. When greeting the interviewer(s), smile, look directly into his or her eyes, and shake hands firmly. After greeting the members of the interview panel, concentrate on appearing pleasant and relaxed. Ask where the interviewer would prefer you to sit. Be conscious of your body language; sit in the "success posture": feet on the floor, shoulders back, and lean in slightly toward the interviewer.

WHAT TO EXPECT? Most interviews begin with a brief discussion related to the weather, traffic, or your travel to the interview site. After the initial greetings, the real interview will begin. This is where your preparation becomes useful. The interviewer(s) will begin to ask you questions related to your strengths, abilities, and qualifications for the job. Listen carefully to the interviewer's question and take time to think about the question and formulate a good answer. If you do not understand the question, ask them to repeat it. Clarify or paraphrase if necessary to be sure you understand. If you do not know the answer, say so. Your answers should be succinct and contain examples whenever possible.

Allow the interviewer to set the tone and pace of the interview. Answer only direct questions, and try not to stray off topic. Be honest in your answers, and be friendly and enthusiastic (Hegarty & Wheeler, 1998). If you go blank during the interview but would like to respond, ask the interviewer if you can think about the question and come back to it in a couple of minutes.

POTENTIAL QUESTIONS YOU MAY BE ASKED. The types of questions you may be asked during an interview are unlimited; however, there are some general questions that are usually asked before more job-specific questions are asked. The samples in the box below represent some possible questions you may encounter during the interview process.

---

### Questions You May Be Asked During an Interview

1. Tell us about yourself, your background, education, and career history.
2. Where do you see yourself in 5 years? What are your long-term career goals?
3. What words best describe you? How would your colleagues describe you?
4. Describe a difficult work situation you have had to deal with. How did you handle it?
5. What are your strengths? What do you see as your areas for development?
6. Why do you want to work for this organization? Why do you want this job?
7. Why should we hire you? How can you make a difference in this organization?
8. What is your philosophy of nursing? What does nursing mean to you?
9. Describe a situation that demonstrates your ability to adapt to changes at work.
10. Describe the best manager/supervisor you have ever worked for. What made them the best?

The type of position for which you are interviewing will determine the specific questions you are asked. However, the sample questions listed in the previous box are quite common. Human rights codes in many jurisdictions prohibit discrimination in employment on various grounds. Questions that may contravene human rights legislation include inquiries about race, religion, age, and marital status. You need to be prepared to answer questions such as this in a way that you feel comfortable. Try to respond in a straightforward and non-aggressive manner.

Questions related to salary are not usually discussed until after a position has been offered. It is worthwhile to have an idea of what the expected salary range is before the interview in case you are asked what you expect. To find out an expected salary range, contact others in the same or similar positions, or check with professional associations or unions, who often have access to such information.

IT IS YOUR TURN TO ASK THE QUESTIONS. The interview is an opportunity both for the employer to get to know you and for you to get to know the employer. It is your opportunity to find out more about the position and the organization to see if it is really something you want. Therefore develop some questions that will allow you to gather information to help decide if this position is what you are looking for. Doing so is particularly important at this time, when organizations are competing globally to recruit nurses. Look for an employer who is willing to help you meet your career goals. The sample questions listed in the box below may be useful in determining your fit with the organization.

---

### Questions You May Ask at an Interview

1. What are the organization's, program's, or department's philosophy and goals?
2. Why is the position vacant?
3. What type of orientation would I receive? What resources will I have access to during my orientation?
4. What are the ongoing opportunities for professional development?
5. To whom would I report? What is your management style?
6. What other health care providers work on this team/service/program? What is the skill mix?
7. What do you think the major challenges of this position will be?
8. What hours would I be required to work? Is there an opportunity to create flexible working hours?
9. What are the next steps in the hiring process? Will there be further interviews? When will the hiring decision be made?

---

The interview allows you to have your questions answered and also lets you see the people with whom you may be working and to see their group dynamics. How they communicate with you and among themselves is a good indicator of what it is like to work with them on a daily basis. Could you see yourself working with this group of people?

When all questions have been answered, the interviewer will bring the interview to a close. Before leaving, thank the interviewer(s) for their time and shake hands as you leave. Be sure they have the necessary information to contact you regarding the hiring decision.

*Follow-Up After the Interview.* A thank you note can be sent by e-mail or handwritten depending on your personal preference. Even if you have decided that you are not interested in the position, you can still express appreciation for being considered. In fact, if you decide that you wish to withdraw your candidacy for the position, it is courteous to let the employer know as soon as possible.

If you have not heard from the employer within the specified time frame, wait a few more days. Then call and ask where they are in the hiring process and whether a decision has been made. With other priorities in the workplace, hiring may be moved down the list. Do not despair or sit and worry; be proactive and get clarification about the new time frame.

*Learning from the Experience.* How did the interview feel? Did you feel confident or unprepared? Each interview situation presents a valuable learning experience. Review the interview. What went well? What would you change for the next time? Make notes to remind you for future interview preparation. If you were unsuccessful in being offered the job, seek feedback from the interviewer if possible. An alternative is to review the interview with a colleague, career coach, or mentor for support and constructive feedback. What can you take from this experience to your next interview?

### Providing References

Employers usually ask for references only after they have determined that you are a final contender for the position. Depending on the position, you will likely be asked to provide three names of people you have worked for or with in the past 5 years. You do not need to use your current manager, especially if you have not advised your current employer that you are searching for alternative work. You can choose a previous employer who will provide you with an excellent reference. The people you choose should be able to enhance the information you provided in the interview. Be sure to get permission from the individuals you list, and contact them to let them know they may receive a call. Describe the position for which you have applied, describe the content of the interview, and review what areas you would like them to highlight when they are called. Give them as much information as possible so they can speak knowledgeably and positively about your abilities.

### The Job Offer

Congratulations! You have been offered the position. Now you need to evaluate the offer and make your decision. The position will likely be offered verbally followed by a written offer. Take your time to review the position description, compensation, and benefits offered. Do not just jump to sign on the dotted line. Look back at your self-assessment and career goals. Will accepting this position help you achieve those goals? Assess the pros and cons of accepting the offer.

There may be some aspects of the job offer that you would like to negotiate (e.g., salary, benefits). If the position is unionized, individual negotiation will not be an option. If it is a non-union position, there may be room for negotiation on some aspects. Be sure you understand what the employer considers by compensation. There may be opportunities to negotiate issues related to education days, vacation, or flex time. To negotiate, you need to know what you want and be prepared to ask for it. Have a couple of scenarios available before discussing them with the employer. If the offer does not feel right, don't accept it. You don't want to regret taking the position in a couple of months. If you refuse the position, do so politely so as not to close the door on future opportunities.

If you were not offered the position, accept the "rejection" letter or phone call in a professional manner. Remember, not every job will be a good fit for you, whether or not it has been offered. Never burn bridges, because another opportunity with this employer may come up in the future.

### Making Presentations

Nurses can use presentations as another strategy to market themselves. Similar to writing for publication, nurses can take the same issues and present on how they have made a difference to patient care or have implemented a new clinical practice, or they can share research findings. There are many opportunities to participate in informal and formal presentations.

Informal opportunities include presenting in your workplace (e.g., conducting an education session for peers or students within your program). It also includes the impromptu teaching nurses do with patients and families on a daily basis. Formal presentations in your workplace could include presenting at patient and nursing rounds or delivering patient education programs.

There are many other opportunities outside your workplace for marketing your skills and knowledge to colleagues and leaders within and outside of the profession. Such forums include professional conferences and workshops through concurrent or poster presentations. If these opportunities seem intimidating, entice a colleague to co-present with you. The more often you present at such events, the more people will get to know you and your expertise. Who knows? This may lead to other career and networking opportunities. A final opportunity to present outside a clinical workplace is through teaching in nursing education programs. Teaching in full-time or part-time capacities provides other means to share your knowledge and expertise.

### Acting as a Mentor

Seeking a mentor may help you achieve your career goals; in the same way, acting as a mentor can help you achieve these goals (Bower, 2000). If one of your goals is to share your knowledge and expertise with other nurses, then why not volunteer to be a mentor? A true mentor-protégé relationship should mutually benefit each party (Fawcett, 2002). While sharing your expertise, you may also benefit by learning from the protégé. Being a mentor may not seem like a self-marketing opportunity, but you will in fact be acting as a role model by sharing your knowledge, skills, and accomplishments with a less experienced nurse.

## CONCLUSION

Self-marketing is about using your various resources to present yourself in the best and most positive way. This chapter has provided you with a variety of strategies and tools for marketing yourself both in writing and in person. To be effective, these tools must incorporate what you learned in your self-assessment and must truly represent who you are and what you have to offer. Creating effective tools (e.g., résumés, cover letters, and business cards) and enhancing your interview skills can create a positive professional image and can give you an edge in your search for rewarding career opportunities. Time is not stagnant, nor is your career. Time and experience will no doubt lead to new career goals and directions. Understanding how to create a self-marketing plan is the key to career success no matter what the stage of your career. Remember, you are your own best resource and cheerleader. You have control over how you present and market yourself to others, both now and in the future.

You now have a thorough understanding of the Model and how to use it. To ensure that you are getting the most out of your career planning activities, you should consider regularly evaluating how your career planning activities are working for you. Complete the questionnaire in Figure 6-8 either after each career change or on an annual basis. Doing so will help you determine which phases of the model need more attention, updating, or consultation and support.

## Scanning
- ☐ I am aware of the current realities and future trends at the global, national, and local level *within* health care and the nursing profession.
- ☐ I am aware of the current realities and future trends at the global, national, and local level *outside* health care and the nursing profession.

## Assessing
- ☐ I can describe my strengths and how I use them in my work.
- ☐ I can describe my limitations.
- ☐ I know how others would describe me.
- ☐ My current position is a good match with my values, beliefs, knowledge, skills, and interests.

## Vision
- ☐ I can describe my ideal vision for my work.

## Planning
- ☐ I can identify my career goals.
- ☐ I have a written career development plan in place.
- ☐ I know what steps to take over the next 6 to 12 months to further my career.

## Marketing
- ☐ I have established a relevant network.
- ☐ I have a mentor or am considering acquiring a mentor.
- ☐ I continue to develop my communication skills through presentations and publications.
- ☐ I have an up-to-date résumé.

Figure **6-8.** How am I doing?

## REFERENCES

Bower, F. (2000). Mentoring others. In F.L. Bower (Ed.), *Nurses taking the lead: Personal qualities of effective leadership* (pp. 255-275). Toronto, Ontario, Canada: Saunders.

Case, B. (1997). *Career planning for nurses.* Toronto, Ontario, Canada: Delmar.

Davis, N. (2001). Writing cover letters with credibility. *Career Planning and Adult Development Journal, 17*(4), 20-28.

Dixson, K. (2001). Every job searcher needs an e-resume. *Career Planning and Adult Development Journal, 17*(4), 66-78.

Enelow, W. (2001). Introduction to this issue. *Career Planning and Adult Development Journal, 17*(4), 4-7.

Enelow, W. (2002). *101 ways to recession-proof your career.* Toronto, Ontario, Canada: McGraw-Hill.

Fawcett, D. (2002). Mentoring-what it is and how to make it work. *AORN Journal, 75*(5), 950-954.

Hacker, L. (1999). *Job hunting in the 21st century: Exploding the myths, exploring the realities*. New York: St. Lucie Press.

Hegarty, L., & Wheeler, M. (1998). The interview: An excellent self-marketing opportunity. In G. Donner & M. Wheeler (Eds.), *Taking control of your career and your future: For nurses by nurses*. Ottawa, Ontario, Canada: Canadian Nurses Association.

Kursmark, L. (2001). Writing effective resumes. *Career Planning and Adult Development Journal, 17*(4), 8-19.

McGowan, R. (2002). Job vs. work: The trend toward nontraditional employment is putting a new spin on conventional careers. http://www.contact.point.ca.

Whitcomb, S.B., & Kendall, P. (2002). *e-Resumes: Everything you need to know about using electronic resumes to tap into today's job market*. New York: McGraw-Hill.

## FURTHER READING

Krannich, R. (2002). *Directory of websites for international jobs*. Lynchburg, VA: Career Masters Institute.

Krannich, R., & Enelow, W. (2002). *Best resumes & CVs for international jobs*. Lynchburg, VA: Career Masters Institute.

Simans, M. (2001). The "p"rinciples of marketing. *The Contact Point Bulletin*, http://www.contactpoint.ca

Watters, M., & O'Connor, L. (2001). *It's your move: A personal and practical guide to career transition and job search for Canadian managers, professionals and executives*. Toronto, Ontario, Canada: HarperBusiness.

# PART II

# Career Planning Throughout Your Career

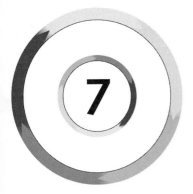

# Career Planning and Development for Students: A Beginning

Janice Waddell, RN, MA, PhD

**Janice Waddell** is an Associate Professor and Associate Director in the School of Nursing, Ryerson University. Janice, who has a special interest in working with students in the career planning process, is also an Associate with donnerwheeler.

## Author Reflections

*Each time I have the opportunity to engage in the career planning and development process with students I am struck by the sense of energy and confidence that students gain through active involvement in the process. They discover so much about themselves, their potential, and their ability to create their professional futures. It is a most rewarding experience to see students take control of their academic and professional careers. Their excitement never fails to reinforce my enthusiasm for nursing and for teaching.*

*Learning without thought is labour lost; thought without learning is perilous.*
***Confucius***

Nurses propose that client discharge planning should begin at the time of admission to the hospital. This philosophy also holds true for career planning strategies for nursing students; the time to begin developing them is the first year of your nursing program. New nursing graduates face a broad range of career opportunities and are challenged to position themselves in a diverse and highly competitive job market. Miller et al. (1984) suggest that, with its variety of career options, nursing has a great deal to offer students who are able to articulate their strengths and who have developed a process of establishing their career goals. Having a clear understanding of one's career objectives—and the skills and knowledge required to attain them—is necessary for a successful job search (Lyon & Kirby, 2000). Starting early is the first step. Allen (1997) advises that it takes times to develop many of the skills and attributes that employers look for in potential employees. Therefore if you can start your career planning process in the early stages of your nursing education, you will enter the job market with a definite advantage (Allen, 1997).

Your nursing program can offer you unlimited opportunities to develop the skills and resources needed to meet career challenges with confidence and enthusiasm. Moreover, the student experience comes with benefits not enjoyed by nurses in the workplace. In your student role, you are exposed to a wide range of clinical settings, you are up-to-date on both theoretical and technological advances, and you have a growing sense of the current issues in the field of nursing and in the health care system as a whole. Classroom and clinical experiences also provide the structure to assist you in developing the adaptive, self-directed learning skills that are important as you create your career (Lyon & Kirby, 2000). You are already ahead of the game! Equipped with some career planning strategies, you can learn to create meaningful and career-enhancing experiences both in the classroom and in clinical settings.

In this chapter you will learn how to adapt the career planning and development process described in previous chapters to meet the particular career planning needs of nursing students so they can appropriately begin what should be a career-long concern. Variants of the environmental scan, self-assessment, reality check steps, career visioning, and self-marketing tips will help nursing students to meet the unique challenges and advantages available to them. Although the focus of this chapter is on students who are not yet registered nurses, registered nurse students may also find aspects of the chapter useful while capitalizing on educational experience as a career development strategy. Nurses who work with students in their clinical placements as mentors or preceptors may also find this chapter helpful.

Students are also referred to the student guide, *Building Your Nursing Career* (2004) for a comprehensive approach to career planning, including guided activities to help master each step of the career planning and development process. In addition to the structured student-focused career planning and development activities, *Building Your Nursing Career* illustrates what career planning looks like "in action" through the stories and suggestions of nursing students themselves. It is a guide you can use throughout your educational program (and beyond) to ensure that your educational experiences help to maximize your future career as a registered nurse.

## WHERE DO I START?

The career planning process involves thought, insight, and dedicated time. Although many resources are available for you to use in planning your career, the one most important resource to your career development is you! Incorporating the career planning process into your approach to your nursing education will help you to develop the knowledge and resources to shape your student experience. Once you have accepted the challenge of career planning, you will be ready to take the first step in the career planning process.

## Scanning the Environment: Making Your Academic and Clinical Environments Work for You

Scanning the environment is something you have already been introduced to as a nursing student. As you learn to plan and deliver nursing care, you also learn to observe your client's environment and the broad range of social, economic, and other variables that influence his or her health status. Meanwhile you also learn about the current trends and issues in nursing, health care, work design, and society at large. The process by which you have gained this knowledge must become part of your ongoing development as a professional. You need to learn to make scanning a continuous and ongoing activity so you can use the information you gained to plan care and to develop your career.

Nursing program goals and outcomes can also provide you with a professional frame of reference to help you focus on broad areas of career development. Broad program goals related to competency in the areas of communication, leadership, knowledge, and professional practice reflect priority requirements for nursing practice and can serve as an excellent guide for your career development activities. Other resources that can provide assistance in determining strengths important to enhance or areas in which to focus your development are nursing and health care-related journals, local and national newspapers, and career advertisements in journals and newspapers. Discussions about current trends in nursing practice and descriptions of skills outlined in job advertisements can offer valuable cues about which nursing skills are considered necessary in the current market. Chapter 2 and *Building Your Nursing Career* offer other suggestions concerning how to scan your environment and also provide you with a practical and up-to-date scan of today's health care environment.

## Completing Your Self-Assessment: Taking Time to Reflect

To develop your career in a way that reflects your values and beliefs, you must have a high degree of self-knowledge (Barner, 1994; Donner & Wheeler, 1998). The self-assessment process assists individuals to reflect on both personal and professional attributes and accomplishments and to look at needs for ongoing professional development. As a student nurse, you also should be aware of the values, skills, strengths, and areas you would like to develop further. You can draw on your work experiences, leisure activities, and other life experiences to help you advance the development of your self-knowledge (Lyon & Kirby, 2000). Such awareness also comes from exploring the reasons you chose nursing as your career and from reflecting on your professional experiences in academic and clinical areas. The insight you gain from your scanning and self-assessment will form the foundation for all your career planning activities. You should begin developing it in the first year of your nursing program.

In many ways students have an advantage in this step of the career planning and development process. Most nursing curricula require that you participate in some form of self-reflection. Students often submit a journal of their reflections about their clinical experiences, including the application of relevant theory to enhance their understanding of their experiences. This reflective process provides an opportunity to become more self-aware by helping you to clarify your values, affirm your strengths, and identify your learning needs in the context of specific clinical experiences. Your increased self-knowledge can help you to broaden your perspective and to see alternatives for your nursing practice (Lauterbach & Becker, 1996). Taking advantage of the support you have for self-reflection in your nursing education will help you to master the process of self-assessment and make it an integral aspect of your career development and your practice.

The questions that registered nurses are urged to ask themselves are also appropriate for you in structuring your approach to your self-assessment. General categories from Chapter 3 are discussed, with suggestions about how student nurses may adapt questions to their situations.

### Values and Beliefs

When you examine how your values and beliefs relate to nursing, it would be helpful for you, as a student, to reflect on why you chose nursing as a career. Ask yourself the following questions (Anderson, 1992; Miller et al., 1984):

1. Were there significant experiences, interests, or skills that prompted you to consider nursing as a career?
2. Was there a nurse you would like to emulate? If so, what qualities did the nurse possess? What values did the nurse convey?
3. What was it about nursing that made you feel that it was a good fit in terms of furthering your interests and skills?
4. What values do you hold that you believe are important for nursing?
5. How will your values influence your learning and your professional development as a nurse?
6. How do you feel that you can contribute to nursing?

The answers to these questions will help you better understand what you are seeking from a nursing career and what aspects of nursing are priorities for you.

As you continue your nursing education, you will need to review your values and interests, adding to them and refining them in response to your growing nursing and personal experiences. It is exciting to watch how your values help you interpret your learning experiences and how your learning experiences influence your values. Self-reflective strategies such as journal entries can help you to keep track of your evolving values, goals, and interests. You can then begin to use your values in a systematic way to evaluate and select possible career paths (Boyatzis, Cowen, & Kolb, 1994). You may also take advantage of the experiences of different faculty members. Asking faculty to share significant events that helped them to clarify their professional values and beliefs can be informative and compelling (Miller et al., 1984).

### Identifying Strengths and Areas for Further Development

Reviewing past accomplishments and nursing program goals are two means of identifying your strengths and the areas you would like to develop further. As you accumulate classroom and clinical experiences, you will also gather feedback from a variety of instructors, peers, and clinical contacts regarding your strengths, your progress, and the areas you need to develop. It is important to reflect on both your strengths and the areas you would like to develop further, so you can both structure and interpret your learning experiences in a way that is relevant and meaningful to you.

If you are in the first year of your basic nursing program, you can start by considering your past accomplishments. Many of the successes and strengths you have enjoyed in other areas of your life will hold you in good stead in your nursing career. Review your past accomplishments with a focus on the values, insight, skills, and strengths you developed as a result of your efforts. Students who have a clear sense of their strengths and skills can focus on enhancing them in the context of their nursing experience by asking for specific feedback and seeking experiences to meet their unique learning needs. Awareness of their values can also add insight and clarity to their reflection and evaluation of each learning experience.

### Using Your Self-Assessment in Your Clinical Placements

The more you learn and reflect on your development as a nurse, the more you can begin to influence and direct your learning experiences. What you learned from your self-assessment can help you to take the initiative to seek out clinical experiences that are congruent with your values, beliefs, and developing skills. Some students enter nursing programs with a clear vision of the area of nursing in which they wish to practice. The self-assessment process provides these students with an opportunity to keep track of the target skills they need to develop to achieve proficiency in their chosen specialty.

In the initial years of most nursing education programs, students are required to complete their clinical placements in organizations that provide experiences in keeping with the general goals of the curriculum. In these settings, students with a definite career goal can still maintain a focus on developing the general practice skills that will be necessary in their future practice specialty. Clinical experiences in diverse settings can also help students to delineate which nursing practice skills are necessary regardless of the clinical setting and which skills are particular to their chosen specialty. In addition to developing relevant clinical skills, students can take time to do some additional research related to their chosen career path. They can interview nurses working in their selected specialty as a means to explore the career opportunities within this practice area.

Of course, many students entering nursing do not have a specific career goal. It is not unusual for them to be uncertain about which experiences would be most beneficial to their professional development. However, if they devote time and effort to reaffirm, discover, or expand their values, strengths, and interests after each clinical experience and academic term, they will be better able to plan for future experiences and to identify their specific areas of interest and aptitude. At the very least, reflecting on experiences and related professional growth offers students information to take to a faculty member or peer for help in clarifying opportunities for further skill development.

## The Reality Check: Validating Your Perceptions

An important aspect of the self-assessment process, the reality check, involves seeking feedback from others. It can be obtained from faculty members, peers, or any other individual whom you trust to offer you an objective and informed response. The reality check is not intended as a means for others to evaluate your self-assessment; instead it is used to confirm the information in your self-assessment and to add a different perspective that may help you refine or rethink parts of it. Individuals often find that the reality check provides an opportunity to be informed (or reminded) of strengths and attributes that they do not recognize in themselves. The reality check component of the self-assessment process can serve to strengthen your confidence in communicating your skills and uniqueness to colleagues, potential employers, and other professionals.

Armed with your regular formal evaluations from instructors, peers, and nursing contacts; your expanding nursing experience; and your initial assessment of your strengths, values, and accomplishments as you enter nursing, you have what you need to update your self-assessment on an ongoing basis.

## Creating Your Career Vision: Daring to Dream

The knowledge you gain from your environmental scan and self-assessment is the foundation from which you can begin to shape your educational experiences to help you meet your career aspirations. Your career vision is the link between who you are and what you can become. Your career vision is less about a specific job and more about recognizing and pursuing your career dreams. Asking yourself "What type of nurse do I want to be?" helps you to start creating your career vision. Your vision can then guide you as you capitalize on and create new learning opportunities.

When you have a vision of what you want your career to look like, you can participate in any course or clinical placement with a sense of how it may help you to get where you want to go. After each learning experience, return to your self-assessment and your vision and ask yourself if both continue to reflect who you are and what you want. Your vision may alter or change dramatically with each new educational experience. The dynamic nature of your career vision does not mean that your initial vision was not right for you at that time, but rather that it is responsive to your ongoing professional growth and development.

Your career vision can focus on a specific practice specialty or, more generally, on your professional identity. Students can use their career vision to guide and motivate them as they participate actively in their academic program. Sharing your vision with your student colleagues, faculty members, and clinical preceptors will allow these supports and resources to help you select and make the best of learning opportunities. As you progress in your nursing program, your vision may become more focused, change, or remain the same. The important thing is that you continue to think about what you want from your nursing career and use it to guide you.

## Your Strategic Career Plan

As you develop and refine your values, skills, and interests related to your nursing practice, you can take advantage of and create opportunities to assist you in achieving your career vision. There are many ways in which you can begin to work toward your career goals. The strategic career plan is really a blueprint for action. It provides you with a process and a structure to help you to work in partnership with your educational supports to achieve your career goals. The strategic career plan helps you to move forward systematically with your plans for further research related to career goals, relevant clinical placement options and related experiences, and the identification of appropriate resources. As with your career vision, you do not need to have a specific clinical specialty in mind for a strategic career plan to work for you. Your career goals follow from your career vision and can be directly related to the areas of development you identified in your self-assessment, such as enhancing communication skills in crisis situations, increasing your involvement in your professional organization, or researching educational opportunities related to clinical skill development. Having a strategic career plan helps you use your career vision to make your related career goals action oriented. You may have more than one strategic career plan at any given time as you explore options related to your career goals.

The strategic career plan you adopt to help you achieve your unique career vision can offer the added advantage of providing you with an opportunity to meet a variety of nurses, and for them to meet you. Each professional encounter you have becomes a chance for you to learn about nursing careers, to express your interest, and to market your growing accomplishments!

## Marketing Yourself in the Academic and Practice Settings

In the context of career planning, marketing simply means that student nurses must not only be clear in their own minds about their strengths and the contributions they can make to professional practice, but they also must be able to communicate that information confidently and effectively to others. This communication can occur in formal interactions with others, in written form, and in informal discussions with professional colleagues. The key to successful marketing is to develop an approach that is congruent with your values and communication style and is true to your abilities. If that congruency is achieved, you are not "selling yourself"; you are asserting your professional strengths and accomplishments in a way that fits with who you are.

Chapter 6 provided you with valuable information and guidance in terms of broader concepts related to the self-marketing process. The following discussion is specifically focused on how nursing students can establish professional networks, benefit from mentoring relationships, build a résumé, and prepare for an interview. *Building Your Nursing Career* provides more depth and specific examples in these areas.

### Networking Within Your School of Nursing

Networking can serve many purposes for nursing students. It involves meeting with a variety of people who share similar interests, practice in areas of nursing that are attractive to you, and can offer you new ideas, perspectives, and opportunities. Besides being a valuable way to establish and maintain your sense of professional identity, networking also offers you the opportunity to inform others of your career vision and your related career goals and activities. Your networking activities will likely become more focused as you progress in your education program. Initially, you may feel unsure about the most appropriate place to begin networking. When you are not ready to choose or are not interested in choosing a specific clinical focus for your nursing career, it may be most beneficial to concentrate your networking activities within your school of nursing and on the contacts that arise as a result of your academic experiences. You can benefit from networking resources in the broader nursing community as you start developing questions related to career options and defining your professional interests. Remember that your ongoing self-assessment and your career vision will also help you to identify specific interests and areas about which you desire further information or development.

At the outset of your nursing education, it is important to discover who your classmates are and how you can establish a sense of involvement in your school of nursing. Your self-assessment and vision will help you to clarify why you are in nursing and what you hope to achieve during your nursing education. Getting to know your student colleagues helps you to meet others with similar goals and interests. It also offers you the chance to find out about interesting courses, clinical placements, and resources—not to mention the support you could enjoy through your interactions with others who are experiencing similar challenges and adjustments.

Faculty members represent another opportunity for networking that is "at your fingertips." Each faculty member has recognized expertise in one or more of the areas of clinical practice, research, and education. As you discover the diversity of nursing practice and start to identify your clinical interests and strengths, you have the benefit of any number of faculty resources for information, guidance, and support. The exchange of ideas can be a mutually rewarding experience for you and the faculty member.

In general, nurses in every realm of nursing enjoy talking about their chosen area of practice and find it reinforcing to see students take an interest in what they do. Faculty members you respect and admire can be excellent resources for you, even if they do not have expertise in the area that interests you. When faculty are aware of students' interests, they can inform them of upcoming events, articles, courses, and opportunities to further professional development. Another benefit of networking with faculty becomes apparent when you require academic references for employment or for admission to subsequent academic programs. Faculty who know you and who have had the opportunity to observe and participate in your professional development are able to provide you with a reference that can clearly reflect your academic accomplishments along with your personal and professional strengths. Finally, faculty can help you to determine the most appropriate and helpful networking resources outside of the academic setting.

### Networking Outside the Educational Setting

Your professional organization offers a wide variety of forums in which you can network with nurses. Joining the professional organization would provide you with the opportunity to participate in any number of interest groups that focus on different aspects and specialties of nursing practice. Many professional organizations also have specific interest groups for students. In addition, general meetings of the organization and meetings of clinical interest groups can offer you the chance to attend educational sessions and to network with nurses practising in various clinical settings. Depending on the focus of your career vision, you can gather helpful information about how best to position yourself to take advantage of opportunities that may become available in specific clinical settings. You may consider asking the following questions of nurses working in specific areas:

1. What do nurses do in that position?
2. What further education would be helpful to gain entry into that field of nursing?
3. Is there a need for nurses in that field?
4. Are there different ways to gain a position in that field?
5. Is there someone specific whom I should meet to discuss my interest in such a position?

Talking to a recent graduate who is working in an area of interest to you may help you to identify issues and strategies unique to new graduates.

Volunteer work also provides rich networking opportunities. Many opportunities in the community can provide valuable and interesting challenges for you, expand your interests, and put you in touch with new people. These opportunities can help you improve your career options in the future. Refer to Chapter 6 for further ideas and strategies about self-marketing in a volunteer position.

### Finding a Mentor

A mentor is someone who takes a personal and professional interest in your professional development. A mentor guides you in that development and seeks out opportunities for you to advance in your nursing career. A mentor is someone you respect and is someone who possesses the professional characteristics to which you aspire. Individuals can have more than one mentor and may have different mentors at various stages in their nursing careers. For nursing students, a mentor may be a faculty member who has taken a special interest in you, has influenced your career decisions, and who helps "open doors" for you.

Not everyone has a mentor; nor is it necessary to have a mentor in your career planning process. However, if there is someone you respect whom you would like to have as a mentor, ask that person if he or she would be willing to act in that role. It is an honour to be asked to be a mentor, but it is important to recognize that mentoring is a responsibility that requires a commitment of time and energy. Respect that commitment by making a formal request of the individual you wish to have as a mentor.

### Preparing for Your Clinical Placement Interviews

Many clinical agencies now require that students participate in an interview before being considered for a clinical placement. You should plan for these interviews as thoughtfully and thoroughly as you would for a job interview.

If your self-assessment, career vision, and strategic career plans are up-to-date and you have done your preparation, your chances of enjoying a successful interview are high. Clear learning goals that are based on your self-assessment, career vision, and nursing program objectives and are customized to the clinical setting will be important to have at the time of the interview. The interview process also represents an opportunity for you to market your strengths and accomplishments. Refer to *Building Your Nursing Career* for a comprehensive guide to preparing for and participating in an interview and for help in preparing for your first job interview—the one you will get right after you graduate.

### The Résumé: Your Written Self-Marketing Strategy

Your résumé is a summary of your skills and accomplishments and is one of your most valuable written self-marketing strategies. A résumé can also serve as a means of monitoring your progress in building the strengths and expertise you have identified in your self-assessment. Cross-referencing your self-assessment and your résumé on an ongoing basis will ensure that you are keeping current in your efforts to develop in your career.

Three unique aspects of a student résumé are the clinical experience summary, the list of selected clinical placements and outcome skills and accomplishments, and the documentation of past working experiences, including summer employment. After each clinical placement or academic term, review your résumé to ensure that it is current and reflects your updated self-assessment. The résumé you develop over the course of your nursing education will grow in proportion to your experiences. As you begin to refine your interests and career goals and start to target specific jobs or agencies, you can customize your résumé to fit the requirements of particular employment opportunities. Always keep a file of your general résumé on disk so you can add to it as you move forward in your career development.

### Your References

Faculty members, mentors, clinical preceptors, part-time and summer job employers, and contacts from volunteer activities can be appropriate sources for references for students. It is important that you select individuals who are familiar with your current level of clinical skill development and recent clinical accomplishments relevant to the practice area. *Building Your Nursing Career* provides more information about selecting appropriate individuals for references.

## CONCLUSION

Numerous choices lie ahead of you. You have the energy, the sense of "time," and the skills to make the most of what is available to you and to create choices that have not been discovered. Career-minded student nurses should emphasize opportunities. Individuals who enjoy rich professional careers are the ones who maintain their curiosity about nursing and the world in general (McBride, 1985). As a fourth-year student advises:

> Often it has been opportunity over the course of my years in nursing school that has prompted changes in my career goals and options. Since opportunity cannot always be planned, all I can do is know myself, my strengths, my interests, and my areas for growth, and be prepared to jump when "opportunity knocks." You must always be a "go-getter." Don't wait for an opportunity to come, go and get it!

However you approach your career development, have fun! "There is a spirit of adventure we should each cling to in orchestrating a career" (McBride, 1995, p. 247). Being positive and active in your nursing education and career development will help you to maintain a sense of optimism about yourself and your profession. That optimism will allow you to be open to exciting opportunities. Good luck!

## REFERENCES

Allen, C. (1997). The job market for '97 grads. *Journal of Career Planning and Employment, 57*(2), 47-50.

Anderson, L. (1992). Reviving your career dream. *Nursing 92, 22*(5), 121-122.

Barner, R. (1994). The new career strategist: Career management for the year 2000 and beyond. *The Futurist, 28*(5), 8-14.

Boyatzis, R.E., Cowen, S.S., & Kolb, D.A. (1994). *Innovating in professional education: Steps on a journey from teaching to learning.* San Francisco: Jossey-Bass.

Donner, G.J., & Wheeler, M.M. (Eds.). (1998). Taking control of your career and your future: For nurses by nurses. Ottawa, Ontario, Canada: Canadian Nurses Association.

Lauterbach, S.S., & Becker, P.H. (1996). Caring for self: Becoming a self-reflective nurse. *Holistic Nursing Practice, 10*(2), 57-68.

Lyon, D.W., & Kirby, E.G. (2000). The career planning essay. *Journal of Management Education, 24*(2), 276-287.

McBride, A.B. (1985). Orchestrating a career. *Nursing Outlook, 33,* 244-247.

Miller, M., et al. (1984). Career planning and professional development: A unique course for nursing students. *Nursing Educator, 9*(3), 40-42.

Waddell, J., Donner, G.J., & Wheeler, M.M. (2004). *Building your nursing career.* St. Louis: Mosby.

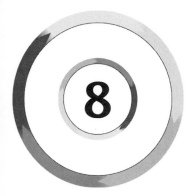

# The Nurse at Mid-Career: What Now?

Mary M. Wheeler, RN, MEd

Mary M. Wheeler, RN, MEd

## Author Reflections

*Considering the question "What now?" has energized me throughout my nursing career. My tenacious curiosity about what could be possible around the next corner, seeing possibilities where no one else can, and then acting on those possibilities have been the cornerstone of my success in nursing.*

*Tell me, what will you do with your one wild and precious life?*

***Mary Oliver***

Recruitment and retention issues are again in the news as health care administrators, policy-makers, nursing organizations, and nurses begin to deal with the reality of a serious shortage of nurses both in North America and around the world. As was discussed in Chapter 2, much attention has been directed toward the need to attract people into the profession, help them see nursing as a lifelong career, and then keep them in nursing. Mid-career nurses currently are the largest cohort in nursing and have the professional memory that employers count on, the expertise patients and clients require, and the experience and wisdom young nurses depend on; however, they are one population at risk for leaving nursing.

These nurses are at mid-career—a point at which they are considering their options within nursing. They are "at a transition period within a career role, at choice points in their career identities" (Carter, 2002, p. 15). They may also be moving toward or have entered mid-life; they are that stage in their personal development where they are stepping back and re-evaluating what is really important in life. This time of renewal and rebirth is a time for "circling back to reclaim dreams and needs that one has lost along the way" (Marston, 2001, p. 4).

This group of nurses, predominantly women, are beginning to examine their own futures after having spent much of their careers and lives caring for others—children, parents, patients. They are often seeking ways to look at their own lives through a different lens, to focus on their needs and their visions for their future rather than on the needs and goals of others. They are asking, "Is that all there is? What has my life been about? What is my purpose? What is the legacy I want to leave?" These questions and their answers are particularly important to the profession at large, which cannot afford to lose these nurses. If these nurses are not helped to rediscover the significance of nursing in their lives and encouraged to see opportunities for further development within the profession, and if options are not made available for them, they can and will choose to leave nursing.

This chapter is directed to those nurses at risk for leaving. It focuses on the uniqueness of nurses at mid-career/mid-life and then, using an adaptation of the Donner-Wheeler Model, provides mid-career nurses with the help they need to navigate this important stage of their careers. This chapter is intended to assist mid-career nurses to re-establish their connection with and commitment to their career and to look at the means to ensure that their career vision and goals are met, either within their current roles and positions or elsewhere.

## WHAT IS MID-CAREER?

The Canadian Institute for Health Information (2001) found that the average age of practising nurses in Canada in 2000 was 43 years—up from 41 years in 1994. During this 6-year period, the percentage of RNs between 50 and 54 years of age who were employed in nursing increased 34% (p. 40). Data from other countries are similar. These changing nursing demographics represent a significant population of nurses who, having established themselves in their careers and personal lives, are now faced with both the challenge and the opportunity to reflect on their career and the meaning it has had for them. Having pursued their education, developed their careers, cared for their families, and given significant energy and a number of years to the health care system, they often find themselves feeling exhausted, depleted, and discouraged. Some begin to question their future within nursing and within health care. Others have no choice in considering their futures, as external forces such as layoffs or restructuring make decisions about their career even more urgent.

Mid-career nurses are at a crossroads and are at a point in their career in which they want to move in a new direction. Mid-career is a time along the career continuum—generally in the consolidation or withdrawal stages (see Chapter 1)—in which one not only steps back and asks the question, "What now?" but also acknowledges that the question needs to be answered. Mid-career has little to do with age or the number of years spent on a given career path; it is marked by shifting career goals for a person who is no longer a beginner in the job (Hall, 1986). Hall found numerous factors indicative of the mid-career experience, including feeling that one's career opportunities are restricted or that there were few opportunities for advancement, becoming aware that personal roles were more important than work roles, and recognizing the relationship between career transitions and life event changes. Fundamental to these experiences is the recognition that one is responsible for one's own career.

Carter (2002) found that women in mid-career have unique developmental needs, including a shifting career identity that emphasizes both achievement needs and a strong desire to remain true to personal definitions of success. Under these expanded definitions, success includes an opportunity to contribute to the community, to develop strong personal relationships with significant others, and to be valued and respected for contributions at work. It is clear that mid-career is a time in which there is a significant opportunity for change and renewal.

## WHAT IS MID-LIFE?

For many, mid-career may also be nested in mid-life. During the first half of life, establishing relationships, families, and careers and attending to the needs of partners, children, and employers have been the priorities. Now we may be faced with possibilities such as divorce, empty nest, elderly parents, grown children, death of a friend, menopause, aging bodies, or illnesses. We question the future much more seriously than in the past. The decisions made in the past were more often than not tied to others and what was best for them. Now we are making decisions about what is best for us. We become more conscious of time marching on, and we do not want to run out of time because we have things left to do. We do not want to have regrets, to look in the mirror one day and say, "I wish I had had more time to...." Because time is of the essence, we are looking more closely at our life, our relationships, and our work.

Mid-life also corresponds with most people's years of highest productivity. The issues of mid-life and work are virtually inextricable. Rohrlich (2001) refers to the Research Network on Successful Midlife Development findings that mid-life is perhaps the least studied and most ill-defined period of any life. It abounds with changing images and myths—the mid-life crisis, the change of life, the empty-nest syndrome, and many more. In the best of cases, people let go and embark on a course of personal reappraisal. They also begin to focus more on the affiliate realm. They join organizations and community groups, creating a legacy in the non-work–related arena.

Awareness of our own mortality surfaces at mid-life and distinguishes this stage from other stages of development. A sense of urgency is created. "It can inspire one to examine what is most meaningful, how one wants to invest their time and energy and enjoy the life that has come to be" (Marston, 2001, p. 11). Issues of advancement, salaries, net worth, higher rungs yet to climb, and continued achievement are questioned by some; the importance of competitiveness recedes and its meaningfulness is questioned.

Many of us have a preconceived notion of mid-life based on our parents' experience. Such ideas can prevent us from seeing this time as full of possibility and potential. Today individuals at mid-life no longer allow themselves to be defined as between youth and old age. They are starting over, motivated to stretch their independence, learn new skills, return to school, plunge into new careers, and rediscover the creativity and adventurousness of their youths and at last listen to their own needs. Sheehy (1995) redefines middle life and concludes: "this is a gift" (p. xvii).

Carl Jung refers to mid-life as the gateway to the second half of life. "We cannot live the afternoon of life according to the program of life's morning, for what was great in the morning will be little at evening, and what in the morning was true will at evening have become a lie" (1933, p. 108). He says that even if the transition is difficult, it is necessary for growth and satisfaction in later life, because growth requires trying out new behaviours and ways of being.

## ISSUES FOR MID-CAREER NURSES

In general, the question "What now?" is asked by mid-life nurses facing mid-career challenges—nurses in their 40s and 50s. Nurses at mid-career tend to ask these types of questions: "Should I go back to school? Should I consider independent practice? Should I take on a leadership role? Should I take a leave? Should I be thinking about retirement? Should I leave nursing?" And for some, "Should I come back to nursing?" Many nurses are looking for the right answers, but most are willing to settle for the right questions.

At mid-career you have a good grasp of nursing work and you are good at it. You also have "different requirements and attitudes to nursing work" (Buchan, 1999, p. 818). You are comfortable in your job, have a great deal of professionalism, and want to reignite the passion about your work. You have or are looking for opportunities to be challenged, professional development support to expand expert competence, broader workplace involvement, flexible work arrangements, and a chance to mentor, teach, and inspire clinical creativity.

With the demands of chaotic workplaces, you may tend to focus additional time on work. As a result, family, friends, community, and self take a back seat. These demands, which result from the changing health care needs of clients, developments in technology, and the shortage of staff, give rise to exhaustion and burnout. Being overly committed to your work, you often feel guilty because the external ideal of caring for others regardless of personal cost has been internalized to the detriment of the need to care for self.

Not only do you have challenges in the workplace, but also you have considerable responsibilities outside the workplace, such as childrearing or providing care to partners, parents, or both. Balancing home and work and staying healthy so that you can provide quality care for clients, family, and yourself becomes a never-ending challenge. The work-life balance and one's ability to achieve it is a popular issue today. We are constantly pursuing this balance, looking over our shoulders and comparing ourselves to others. Moses (2002) asks the question, "Is the solution really to find a better balance? It may be that the whole concept of work-life balance tends to obscure what we're really looking for, namely the opportunity to feel good about our lives and to have a sense of accomplishment" (p. C1).

Many financial realities also present themselves at mid-career, particularly in supporting children in their educational endeavours. Therefore the dream of "freedom 55" may no longer be realistic. Breaks in service and periods of non-contribution to pension schemes will be a factor in determining the retirement behaviours of some nurses who do not have access to other sources of financial support. Buchan (1999) concludes that the need to enhance pension funds and maintain financial stability is likely to be a main reason why many nurses work beyond the 55 years of age. The reality for many of us at mid-career is that we may still be working for some time, and more than likely at our current place of employment.

These are but a few of the numerous issues confronting the mid-career nurse. Each individual will react in various ways to all of these internal and external challenges, from being disgruntled to being curious about the future. Curious nurses recognize that they have possibly 10 to 15 years left to practice and ask themselves what to do with those years so they will be satisfied. Thus asking the question "What now?" clearly differentiates them from others who just go through the motions and are content to let events determine their future. The curious and proactive mid-career nurse chooses a future by design, not drift. The inevitable next step for a nurse at mid-career—whether 38 years old and pondering returning to school, 45 years old and deciding whether to stay in nursing, or 52 years old and realizing the need for an enriched personal life—is to acknowledge that the responsibility for attaining insight and generating change for her career rests primarily with her.

Gros says that "the power to heal, grow, change, and develop comes out of the work that people do themselves. It comes through the actions they take, the choices and decisions they make" (2001, p. N16). Acknowledging that the "self" is significant, important, valuable, and worthy leads one to understand that the need to care for oneself can be found in answering the question, "What now?" Beginning to think about how to answer this question is like beginning a journey.

## THE JOURNEY

*The true journey of discovery does not consist in searching for new territories, but in having new eyes.*

*Proust*

The need to step back and contemplate the question "What now?" resonates for many nurses at mid-career. How to go about answering the question is the challenge. Taking the time to focus on self is a unique opportunity that many nurses do not do often enough—regardless of where they are on the career continuum. All of us at one time or another hear the call. For some it may be a nudge, for others it is a push to answer the question "What now?" Yet not all of us answer the call, the call to do, to be, to move toward something or away from something, or to change something. "Saying yes to the call places you on a path that half of you thinks does not make sense, while the other half of you knows your life won't make sense without" (Levoy, 1997, p.4)

Answering the question "What now?" requires leaving your daily roles, responsibilities, and the business of ordinary life behind and retreating to a space that offers solitude and simplicity. You also need to be open to possibilities. Only after this journey can a new beginning be realized. "Allowing oneself to be vulnerable, defenseless, and non-judgmental and open to totally unexpected options and opportunities is the essence of true exploration, both inner and outer. Freeing yourself from prejudice and preconceptions and embracing serendipity and uncertainty is by far the most effective way of releasing the inner you" (Yeadon, 1996).

Retreat, reflect, renew, and re-enter are the guiding principles for your journey. These guiding principles are what some call "sacred patterns" and are what Levoy describes as when "we leave an old life behind, experience a life transition up close, and receive its thorny wisdom, and then head home and hope to follow through on whatever we learned" (p. 147). As you begin your journey you may feel a mixture of fear, anxiety about the unknown, and guilt related to taking time for yourself. You need to let go and engage in a process of self-reflection and renewal, giving yourself permission to look honestly at who you are and what you want. This will require you to spend time by yourself, listen to yourself, and allow yourself the time to put into perspective what is important in your life.

The optimal setting for this journey is one that allows you to slow down, take smaller steps, and look around; it is a setting in which you are free to wander and discover who you are, what life is about, and what you want from life at mid-career. In such a setting, you can move from action to stillness, from doing to being, and from an outward focus to an inward one. These factors are essential before any inner journey of discovery can occur. You are also encouraged to use journal writing and drawing to document your personal discoveries throughout the process; these are the resources for reflection that you can carry back with you as you re-enter your everyday world. The journal functions more as a place to think than as a tool to use in any explicit way. Your journey is also an opportunity for you to use that creative side of your personality—that part of us we often ignore to focus on the practical aspects of our lives. Creativity can be expressed in an entire range of activities, including drawing, painting, sculpting, dancing, and singing. Neubauer (2000) thinks that nurses overuse words and make greater use of their left brains to the detriment of creativity and intuition. "The arts help people access their creativity and get beyond words, they help people clarify their goals and visions and get to the essence of what they are thinking about" (p. 5). As you contemplate the question "What now?," play with some form of art medium to express, in ways other than words, the multitude of possible answers to this question. To ensure that you stay on the path, a compass is a necessary tool for your journey.

## The Compass

To navigate your journey and to answer the burning question "What now?," you need a compass—a series of questions to refer to when you feel lost or need direction along the way. Levoy says the "questioning is a prerequisite to change and innovation, and without it there is no discovery" (p. 151). Questions shape our lives and often can have more then one answer. Our compass (Figure 8-1), which can take you anywhere you want to go, leads you to your destination in four stages: self-discovery, vision crafting, grounding the vision, and return to community. Self-discovery asks two key questions: "Where have I been?" and "Where am I now?" Vision crafting asks the following questions: "Where would I like to go?" and "What road blocks have the potential to inhibit my journey?" Grounding the vision asks the question, "How will I get there?" Return to community asks, "How will I know I have reached my destination?"

As in any career planning and development activity, the process is iterative, not linear. We encourage you to read the questions asked in the following

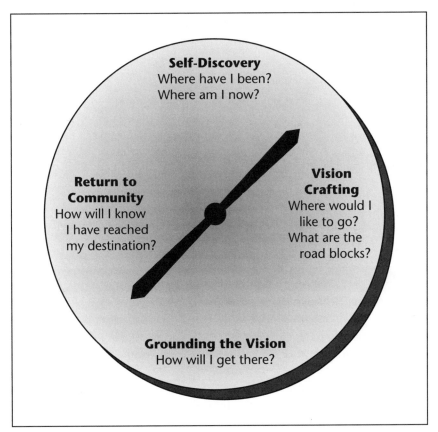

Figure **8-1.** The compass.

sections and reflect on those that have meaning for you. As you begin to read the questions, you may find you are not ready to answer them. Other priorities present themselves. Distractions can be a respite from the harsh task of self-examination. Don't worry. You need to find the right time for you, but you also need to decide that you want to go. Deciding to go can result in amazing journeys.

### Self-Discovery

*Where Have I Been?* We are complex human beings and are the sum of our past and current experiences, both personal and professional. Who we are is like looking at a quilt, rich in colours and designs. This quilt shows where we have been and where we are now. As our self continues to unfold, new experiences are sewn into the ever-growing design. With self-discovery you begin to recognize common themes and patterns that have shaped who you are and what you do. Begin with the question "Where have I been?" Your answers to this question come from mapping your life's journey, as shown in the box below. Start with reflecting on your childhood.

---

### ◄ Reflecting on My Childhood ►

Think back to your early life as a young child. Now ask yourself the following questions:

- Who was that child?
- What was my favourite thing to do as a child?
- What was I most often doing when I lost track of time?

---

Write down in your journal or draw a picture of what comes to mind. If you are finding it hard to remember, talk to your parents, brothers, or sisters. What do they remember about you? What did they think you were good at? Sometimes the first things we are great at are the talents that we carry through our lives.

Next draw a lifeline representing the last 20 years of your life and plot the most significant highlights or milestones in your life, both the highs and the lows (see the box below).

---

### ◄ Examining My Lifeline ►

Look at your lifeline and ask yourself the following questions:

- When did I feel most alive, energized, committed, fulfilled?
- Can I describe those times in my life when I made a difference?
- What three adjectives would others use to describe me and why?

---

*Where Am I Now?* Who you are includes your beliefs and values, your knowledge and skills, and your interests. Two things, being good at something and loving it, tend to go hand in hand. Answering the question "Where am I now?" will help you identify areas in which there is a lack of congruence between who you are and what you do. This is the first step on the path to painting a picture of where you might like to be in the future. See Figure 8-2 and the boxes below.

---

### How Do I Spend My Time?

Look at Figure 8-2. Mark the percentage of time you spend in each section of the circle.

Now ask yourself the following questions:

- Is what I value reflected in the time I spend on each section?
- If not, what aspects would I like to change so there is more congruence between what I value and what I am doing?

---

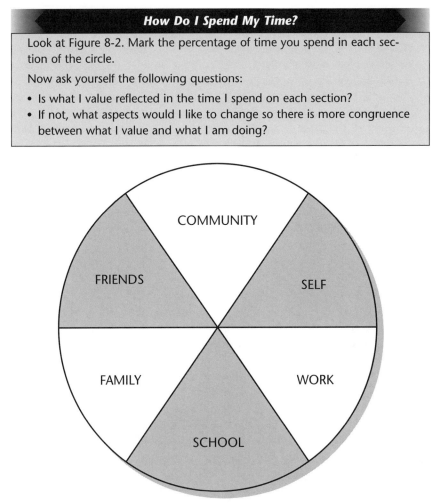

Figure **8-2.** What are my priorities?

---

### What Do I Like to Do?

In your journal, make a list of five things you like to do. Now ask yourself the following question:

- When was the last time I did one of these five things?

If it has been some time since you did things that you like to do, spend some time reflecting on what has happened along the way. Now consider the characteristics that contribute to your uniqueness. See the box below for some questions to help you with this.

---

### My Skills and Talents

In your journal, make a list of your special talents and qualities. Then answer the following questions:

• What gives meaning to my life?
• What am I passionate about?
• Where do I still want to grow?

---

Your answers to the two key questions "Where have I been?" and "Where am I now?" will begin to give you more depth of colour and definition of design to the quilt that is you. In moving through self-discovery you are honouring *what is*. In vision crafting you focus on *what could be*. Having a better understanding of who you are will help in the transition to the next phase of the process, which is answering the question "What do I want?" This is where the fun begins.

### Vision Crafting

*Where Would I Like to Go?* Vision crafting is your brainstorming opportunity, the chance to do some blue sky thinking. Close your eyes so you can connect more easily with your imagination and creativity. Don't worry about your vision being too big, too vague, or too impossible. It should be grand, inspiring and, if it is an important dream, perhaps a little scary (see the boxes below and on p. 115).

---

### What Are My Hopes and Dreams?

Ask yourself the following questions:

• What do I want? What am I seeking and why?
• How do I want to live my life and have my work be a part of my life?
• How can I combine my skills and talents with my dreams?
• If I had 20 times more courage, what would I do?

---

---

### What Is My Vision?

After you have had some time to savour those questions in the box on p. 114, you should be ready to provide more focus as you begin to create your career vision and your ideal vision for your work. Ask yourself the following questions:

- What does this ideal vision look like? What am I doing? Where am I located? Who is around me? How have I structured it?
- What are the values by which I operate?
- What talents and gifts am I using/expressing?
- Is my vision clear, focused, defined?

---

### What Might Inhibit My Journey?

At this juncture you may be saying to yourself, "I want to (fill in your own response), but I can't because (fill in your own response)." It is important to clarify why you feel this way. Many of us believe that we cannot do what we really want to do. It may be that we walk away from our dreams afraid that we may fail or, worse, yet that we may succeed. If you are afraid of something, try to understand what it is and why it scares you.

Ask yourself the following questions:

- What is getting in the way of me becoming what I desire? Why am I stuck in certain ways? Are there external and internal constraints (i.e., external to me [caused by others] vs. internal to me [coming from within myself, ones I create for myself]) that I must consider before I can do what I really want to do?
- What could I do to overcome these external and internal barriers? What steps do I need to take right now?

---

A first step is to go back to your journal and review your accomplishments under self-discovery. The knowledge and skills you used to achieve those accomplishments are the same attributes you will need to use to realize your new vision for your career.

What is it that needs doing that you know something about, that probably will not happen unless you take responsibility for it? Where can you make a difference? You should now be able to describe in your journal what you have created or started to create. This is also a good time to start sharing your vision with others and to let them hear your answer to the question "What now?" Your answer begins with "I am...."

### Grounding the Vision

*How Will I Get There?* You have two strong allies to help you ground your vision: (1) your dissatisfaction with how things have been, and (2) your belief that you can achieve the future you have envisioned for yourself. Your enemies are in responses such as "Why bother?" "It isn't so bad the way it is," "I don't have time," or "I can never have what I want." See the box below.

---

#### Making My Vision a Reality

Begin by walking into that future you have envisioned for yourself as you now ask yourself the following questions:

- How do I create this career vision?
- What inner resources can I tap? What external resources do I need, and from whom? What skills do I need to acquire?
- What will be my first step?

---

*Return to Community.* How will you know you have reached your destination? The return to the "community" can be fraught with difficulties (Galland, 1994). Joseph Campbell (cited in Galland, 1994) put it well: "It's easy enough to go off on a quest but to return—well that's another story. What has been gained can still be lost at this point" (p. 249). Your transition back to reality can be either smooth or rocky. The career vision you have articulated for yourself may take you in a completely new direction from where you were when you began this process. Just taking the risk to embark on this journey and reflect on the questions will give you more insight into the question "What now?" You will need to defend the insights you gain against all those "voices"—both yours and others—that can quickly squash your enthusiasm for what could be. What support and feedback will you need, and from whom, when you re-enter your day-to-day world?

Establishing a support group within your life might be a strategy. This "dream support team" is there on the sidelines as you take steps toward your vision. It is an opportunity to speak and be heard—to discuss with others your struggles, fears, dreams, and discoveries by both naming and describing these experiences. What becomes evident is that you are not alone and that you can make your needs known to others. The more we tell others what we want and what we need from them, the easier it is for them to help us achieve our career goals. Being in a small group, spending time together, and having a shared goal contribute to listening to each other and bonding, thus giving authority to the speaker and his or her ideas. For all of us, the power of shared intention is significant.

Perhaps a more formalized follow-up period, through individual coaching, would be beneficial for you. If you are contemplating a significant career or personal change, a continuous coaching relationship can help you "keep on track." Nurses have not had experience with individual coaching as a way to add value to their lives. The idea that "I can do it on my own" is not unfamiliar to the profession. For nurses who are used to providing guidance and help for others, needing help ourselves is sometimes difficult to acknowledge. Keep asking yourself, "What will it feel like to have realized my career vision?" Levoy (1995) says that you change on your journey and that your vision follows you back and must be incorporated into your life and the lives of those you know. "Vision, if it is anything, is your life story in action" (p. 162).

## CONCLUSION

"The time has come for the individual to begin his true adult education, to discover who he is and what life is about. What is the secret of the 'I' with which he has been on such intimate terms all these years yet which remains a stranger?" (Smith, 1958, p. 64). Mid-career nurses need to find the time and the place in which they are free to discover who they are and what life is about. They need to reflect on "I" in relation to their careers. Moving through the process we have provided in this chapter can make a difference for those mid-career nurses who decide to break free, take a risk, and start answering the all-important question about their professional lives, "What now?"

## REFERENCES

Buchan, J. (1999). The "greying" of the United Kingdom nursing workforce: Implications for employment policy and practice. *Journal of Advanced Nursing, 30,* 818-826.

Canadian Institute for Health Information. (2001). *Canada's health care providers.* Ottawa, Ontario, Canada: Author.

Carter, T. (2002). The importance of talk to midcareer women's development: A collaborative inquiry. *The Journal of Business Communication, 39,* 55-91.

Galland, C. (1994). A new generation of women in the wilderness. In E. Cole, E. Erdman, & E. Rothblum (Eds.), *Wilderness therapy for women* (pp. 243-258). New York: Haworth Press.

Gros, C. (2001). Nurses urged to become the evangelists for self-care. (May 7). *The Globe and Mail,* p. N16.

Hall, D. (1986). Breaking career routines: Midcareer choice and identity development. In D.T. Hall and Associates (Eds.), *Career development in organizations* (pp. 120-159). San Francisco: Jossey-Bass.

Jung, C. (1933). *Modern man in search of soul.* New York: Harcourt, Brace, Jovanovich.

Levoy, G. (1997). *Callings: Finding and following an authentic life.* New York: Three Rivers Press.

Marston, S. (2001). *If not now, when? Reclaiming ourselves at midlife.* New York: Time Warner.

Moses, B. (2002). Forget balance: Focus is the key. (October 2). *The Globe and Mail,* p. C1.

Neubauer, J. (2000). Self-development and the arts. *Creative Nursing, 4,* 5-7, 14.

Rohrlich, J. (2001). Employees at midlife: Crisis or transition? *Business and Health, 19,* 17-21.

Sheehy, G. (1995). *New passages: Mapping your life across time.* New York: Ballantine Books.

Smith, H. (1958). *The religions of man.* New York: Mentor Books.

Yeadon, D. (1996). To go adventuring. *Sojourns, Fall/Winter.*

## FURTHER READING

Belenky, M.F. (1997). *Women's ways of knowing.* New York: Basic Books.

Brook, P. (1997). *Work less, live more.* Toronto, Ontario, Canada: Doubleday Canada Ltd.

Gilligan, C. (1993). *In a different voice.* Cambridge, MA: Harvard University Press.

Hall, D.T., & Mirvis, P.H. (1995). The new career contract: Developing the whole person at midlife and beyond, *Journal of Vocational Behavior, 47,* 269-289.

Jones, M. (1995). *Creating an imaginative life.* Berkeley, CA: Conari Press.

Marmoreo, J. (2002). *The new middle ages.* Toronto, Ontario, Canada: Prentice Hall.

Walker, J. (2000). *Making the most of your midlife career transition.* New York: The Berkeley Publishing Group.

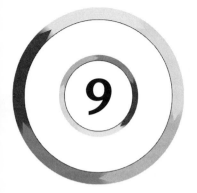

# Creating Career Success Through Entrepreneurship

Michelle Cooper, RN, MScN

**Michelle Cooper** is President of Integral Visions Consulting Inc., a consulting firm that is dedicated to promoting, improving, and sustaining the effectiveness and health of organizations. Michelle launched her business in 1998. She provides consultation and facilitation services and workshops that foster commitment, creativity, enthusiasm, community building, and goal achievement. She is also an Associate with donnerwheeler.

## Author Reflections

*When I think about becoming an entrepreneur, I realize that actively seeking new and challenging opportunities within my employment settings was key to my success. I developed an incredible breadth of knowledge and skills, the courage to take risks, and a belief in myself that makes anything I dream a possibility!*

*If you want to walk on water, you've got to get out of the boat.*

*Ortberg*

The secret to career success is to act as a free agent, accepting responsibility for seeking out or creating opportunities to grow and develop early enough to be able to take full advantage of them in a timely and meaningful way (Manion, 2001; Porter-O'Grady, 1997). The second millennium has brought accelerated rates of change, advancements in knowledge generation and management, advancements in technology, and a concomitant shift in how health care services are organized. Nurses are ideally positioned to positively influence the evolving health care system and to make a difference in the lives of not only the people that we serve, but also those in our communities, countries, and world.

Whole systems changes have created many opportunities for nurse entrepreneurs to apply their skills in independent practice in a variety of areas. However, nurses do not need to leave their places of employment to influence change. Enlightened organizations that understand the need to develop the capacity to lead and manage change from within can provide nurse intrapreneurs with an opportunity to test their entrepreneurial skills within the safety net provided by employment.

This chapter will assist you in developing a business idea or innovative project using the Donner-Wheeler Model. After defining the concepts of entrepreneurship and intrapreneurship, each phase of the Model is reviewed, with a focus on the elements that are specifically or uniquely applicable to entrepreneurship and intrapreneurship. As you proceed, you are encouraged to review the detailed descriptions of each phase covered in previous chapters.

## ENTREPRENEURSHIP AND INTRAPRENEURSHIP

Entrepreneurs are individuals who perceive or create an opportunity to apply their skills and talents and who create an organization to pursue the idea while assuming all of the risks and responsibility for the success or failure of the service or product (Manion, 1990; Orga, 1996). Entrepreneurship involves all of the functions, activities, and actions associated with being an entrepreneur (White and Begun, 1998). Pinchot (1986) coined the term *intrapreneur* to refer to an individual who initiates innovation and applies entrepreneurial skills *within* an organization. Intrapreneurship refers to the functions, activities, and actions of the intrapreneur. The purpose and functions of entrepreneurs and intrapreneurs and the qualities they need to succeed are similar; it is only the context that differs. Entrepreneurs work from the outside to create their own organization, whereas intrapreneurs work from within the organization (Manion, 2001; Porter-O'Grady, 1997).

Nurse entrepreneurs function in a variety of practice settings, such as independent practitioners in sole proprietorships or in partnerships or as presidents and CEOs of their own large corporation. Some have started enterprises that include traditional and complementary nursing care services such as intravenous therapy, occupational health services, foot care, lactation consultation, weight management, healing touch, and wellness consultation. Others provide education such as skills-based workshops, in-services for small health care facilities, or personal development such as career planning. Nurses are also applying their skills to promote health and effectiveness as consultants to organizations within health care and beyond.

Both entrepreneurs and intrapreneurs have the ability to match their skills and passion to an opportunity:

> Connie had a dream of providing a work environment for nurses that was flexible and personally rewarding while providing a valuable health care service. She actively pursued her dream and started up a home health care company. Her company has grown from a small organization with a few nurses serving a focused client group to a large, multi-site corporation with several million dollars in annual revenue that now provides a broad range of interdisciplinary services. The growth was fuelled by her entrepreneurial spirit and continuous seeking of new opportunities.

Nurses have made a difference within their organizations by applying their expertise in innovative and creative new ways. This includes new or better ways to provide care, ideas for new roles or programs, and innovative partnerships with other service providers to organize care delivery:

> Nurse educators in a hospital facing a budget crisis saw an opportunity to market their skills and education programs to smaller long-term care facilities that did not have the budget to hire their own educators. This was a win-win situation that enabled the hospital to retain its expert educators and gave other long-term care facilities access to a range of expertise they would never have been able to afford to develop themselves.

In the last two decades the role of entrepreneurship has assumed greater importance for the individual, the organization, and the profession (White & Begun, 1998). Entrepreneurial skills are emerging as basic job expectations for succeeding in careers inside, outside, or at the margins of the profession. Organizations are recognizing that they need to tap into the potential and encourage the entrepreneurial skills of their employees if they are to attract and retain the very best, as well as to survive and thrive in the future. Entrepreneurship is also a way to advance and energize the profession of nursing by developing innovative roles and practice settings that actively promote the knowledge and skills that nurses bring to the health care sector.

## Rewards and Challenges

It takes courage to be an entrepreneur or an intrapreneur, but it is worth the risk. There are both rewards and challenges. The biggest risk is making the decision to pursue your passion and ideas. The hardest step is the first step.

Figure 9-1 compares and contrasts the rewards and challenges of being an entrepreneur or intrapreneur as identified by a number of authors. The key differences are the freedom to create and the degree of risk. The entrepreneur has complete creative control and assumes full responsibility for developing and implementing the service or product. Intrapreneurs share the risk of their innovations with their organizations. Those who have success with intrapreneurship find great personal reward by staying within organizations. For others, intrapreneurship is a way to build the confidence and skills that lead the way to entrepreneurship. The career paths of most successful nurse leaders and entrepreneurs are built on the foundation of successful intrapreneurship and innovation within health care organizations (Manion, 2001).

Intrapreneurs and entrepreneurs alike can enjoy the benefits of success by learning to identify and manage the potential barriers. Applying the phases of the Donner-Wheeler Model to your business idea or innovation is one way to help you plan for success. As stated in Chapter 1, application of the model is not a linear process. You may find yourself going back and forth between phases as you clarify your idea and goals, increase your self-knowledge, and obtain more data. Planning does not end with the launch of the service, product, or innovation. In fact, it is just the beginning of the next level of planning to ensure that your idea or service constantly adapts to the changing environment or marketplace and is still aligned with your skills and passion.

| | Entrepreneur | Intrapreneur |
|---|---|---|
| **Rewards** | • Control over your work life<br>• Satisfaction—doing what you love<br>• You can't be laid off<br>• Creative license<br>• Profitability—you benefit from the success<br>• More flexible lifestyle<br>• Personal growth and development<br>• An opportunity to influence change on a broader basis | • Shared risk taking—you still have a regular paycheque<br>• Marketing advantage—you have an established reputation in the organization<br>• Access to a broad network of trusted colleagues and to information<br>• Access to professional development opportunities<br>• Personal satisfaction seeing ideas come to life<br>• Feedback and recognition |
| **Challenges** | • Risk of business failure<br>• Time investment—takes long hours to make it work and sometimes years to be profitable<br>• Unpredictable income<br>• Total responsibility for errors, complaints, etc.<br>• Pressure to please customers, creditors, and yourself<br>• Responsibility for getting, doing, and sustaining your own work<br>• Isolation<br>• Competition | • Getting acceptance for ideas within a larger bureaucracy<br>• Smaller organizations may not have the financial assets to support change<br>• Moving ideas from conception to reality takes longer<br>• Frustration at attempts to make changes<br>• Instability and constant restructuring in the health care sector—innovation becomes obsolete before it has life<br>• Ownership of innovation |

Figure **9-1.** Rewards and challenges of being an entrepreneur or intrapreneur. (Modified from Manion, J. [1990]. *Change from within. Nurse intrapreneurs as health care innovators.* Chicago: American Nurses Association; Orga, J. [1996]. *Becoming a nurse entrepreneur.* Tennessee Nurse, 59[2], 13-14; Porter-O'Grady, T. [1997]. *The private practice of nursing: The gift of entrepreneurialism. Nursing Administration Quarterly,* 22[1], 23-29.)

You need to be willing to reinvent your business or innovation or create a new one to stay ahead of the changing needs and demands. You are invited and encouraged to write down your insights in a journal as you go through the phases of the Model. All of the information you gather will eventually be recorded as you develop your business plan.

## SCANNING THE ENVIRONMENT: WHAT ARE THE POSSIBILITIES?

In Chapter 2 you learned in detail how, when, and why to scan the environment as part of your career planning process. Scanning the internal and external environments increases your awareness and conscious "seeing" of the strengths, weaknesses, opportunities, and gaps (Parker, 1998). Scanning in concert with your self-assessment can be the source of an idea for an innovation or enterprise or can help you to clarify it. Once the idea takes shape, scanning becomes a planned and systematic activity as part of a market analysis to determine the validity of and demand for the product or service you plan to offer. For example, in Chapter 2 we learned that shortened lengths of stay are a feature of the new health care system. We also learned that the shift to community-based services is underway. These trends could be seen as opportunities for entrepreneurship.

### Learning from Your Scan

Once you have gathered data from your scan, it is time to analyze it to see if there is an opportunity that fits your skills. Consider the following questions: Are there unmet needs now or anticipated in the future? What would be the best way to meet these needs? Are you interested in meeting these needs? Is anybody else meeting these needs? Are there trends, legislation, or new knowledge that will change the way health services are delivered? Is there something you could do within your organization to address these trends? Does this create opportunities for independent practice? Once you have an idea that you think is a business opportunity, you can validate the idea through a more extensive scan of needs, wants, and demands. This process is described in the next section.

Scanning helped Connie to develop the concept for her business:

> Connie listened to her colleagues talk about the need for more flexibility and control over their worklife. She also knew from experience that there were unmet needs for fragile paediatric clients in the community. That gave her a starting point to begin more systematic research about the viability of starting a private enterprise that would meet both needs. She would provide a work environment that enables staff to flourish and provide the excellent care required for this paediatric group of clients.

The nurse educators found that by looking at the gaps in the community, they could pursue some important activities outside their organization:

The nurse educators heard about the increasing acuity of residents in long-term care facilities and the gap in educational support to meet these needs through a meeting of a local chapter of their Gerontological Nurses Association. At the same time, the staff newsletter identified financial shortfalls and pending restructuring in their organization. Understanding both the opportunity and threat together stimulated their imaginations and provided a potential solution that would help their hospital, the educators, and the broader community.

Scanning the culture and structure of the organization for receptivity to innovation is an important added element for the intrapreneur (Parker, 1998). Does the structure of your organization support intrapreneurship? Does the culture value intrapreneurial spirit? How successful have others been at introducing change? Where does decision-making authority rest? These questions are not meant to discourage the intrapreneur, but instead are meant to help identify potential roadblocks so that strategies for overcoming them can be built into the plan.

Great ideas happen when wonder and imagination come together. Feed your imagination with a variety of rich and diverse information, and take the time to reflect on what you can do within your organization or as an entrepreneur to make the difference you want to make.

### Determining Gaps: Needs, Wants, and Demands

Developing a successful innovation or business venture requires assessment of the needs, wants, and demands of your potential customers. Needs are actual or perceived gaps between what people value or require and what they have that requires an intervention. Wants are satisfied by specific goods or services. For example, home health care services for personal care may be a need. Delivery by a specific professional (e.g., registered nurses rather than non-regulated service providers) may be wanted. Demand occurs when people are willing and able to participate in an exchange of goods or services (Alward & Camuñas, 1991).

Market research is used to understand your customers and to help you to identify, assess, and respond to their needs and wants. The market research process is similar to any other applied research process: Identify the marketing issue and develop a research question, define research objectives, collect data, analyze and interpret data, and communicate the results. The services of professional market researchers can be purchased if you do not have the skills or the resources to complete your own, but this will increase the cost and time needed and may affect the applicability of the data. Marketing students at your local university or college may conduct the research for far less cost as part of a school project.

Now that you have scanned your environment and have an idea that you think you want to pursue, it is time to ask the following question: "Do I have the knowledge, skills, and ability to make this happen?"

## SELF-ASSESSMENT: DO I HAVE THE RIGHT STUFF?

*Three things are extremely hard: steel, a diamond and to know one's self.*
**Benjamin Franklin**

You now need to assess your strengths accurately and honestly to determine whether you have the knowledge and skills to breathe life into your initiative. Getting to know yourself better is the most important step of the planning process. The ability to match your skills to an opportunity is a critical success factor for the entrepreneur and intrapreneur (Porter-O'Grady, 1997):

Connie was able to bring project management experience and excellent communication skills, among others, to her entrepreneurial initiative; the nurse educators were able to apply their expert knowledge of older adults and their program design skills to the intrapreneurial project.

In addition to the information in Chapter 3, a number of self-assessment tools are available in books and on the Internet. These tools can be used to determine the personal strengths and learning needs that you bring to the entrepreneurial table. Some of the attributed skills that researchers have linked to successful entrepreneurs or intrapreneurs are discussed in the following sections.

### Personal Qualities, Knowledge, and Skills

Successful entrepreneurs are highly motivated and have the courage to take the risk, share their ideas, and expend the time, money, and effort to make their dreams a reality (Schneider, 1997; Czaplewski, 1999). They have active imaginations and the ability to translate their dreams into action. Successful entrepreneurs need a mix of personal, leadership, and business skills (Manion, 1990). The degree to which the skills are important depends on the type of business being developed by the entrepreneur and on the organizational supports available to the intrapreneur.

Personal qualities include assertiveness, self-confidence, self-directedness, self-motivation, a high internal locus of control, excellent negotiation skills, flexibility, the ability to deal with uncertainty and ambiguity, and the ability to adapt to change. As innovators, entrepreneurs are change agents and need to have strong leadership skills, be excellent communicators, and have the ability to articulate a vision and to motivate and coach others. Practical management skills such as meeting facilitation, delegation, and project management are also desirable. Above all, implementing change requires perseverance, high energy, and stamina to withstand the inevitable negative or restraining forces that appear when change is introduced (Manion, 1990; Parker, 1998; White & Begun, 1998).

Entrepreneurs require the right credentials and "hard skills," the knowledge and skills relevant to the service or innovation. In general, individuals with an entrepreneurial spirit are proactive in seeking education and professional development opportunities that position them well to seize opportunities. Entrepreneurship is as much an attitude as it is a skill. It requires that individuals take full responsibility for their career success and actively pursue the opportunities and learning experiences that support their dreams to become reality. Confidence in oneself and a passion for one's ideas are the two most important critical success factors.

## Business Skills

Sound business planning, financial management, and marketing skills are important for entrepreneurs. Developing business acumen is often a focus for professional and skill development. Some of the business knowledge and skills required include proposal writing, business plan development, income and expense forecasting, budgeting, and marketing. Entrepreneurs may also require human resource management and other business skills specific to their business (e.g., case management, logistics). Intrapreneurs have the advantage of assistance from within their organizations to learn business skills and to get help in developing the business aspects of an innovation being introduced.

Entrepreneurs need to understand the legal requirements for starting and operating a business. As with any business, an independent nursing practice must comply with local, regional, and federal laws, including licensing and taxation. Nurses must also consider their professional regulations, codes of conduct, and standards of practice. Each jurisdiction has defined the scope of practice for regulated professions. You need to ensure that your product or service fits within your scope of practice, or you need to build the appropriate supports into your structure to enable you to perform your service. If you do not have or cannot obtain the skills you need in the short term, then you can build a team of people around you who can both support you and teach you as you move through the planning and implementation phases.

## Resources and Supports

Understanding your strengths and limitations will help you to identify the resources and support networks you will need. Although the intrapreneur and entrepreneur do have some common needs, there are additional considerations for the entrepreneur. Entrepreneurs must obtain these supports independently and invest time and energy in building and maintaining their support network. In contrast, the intrapreneur has a built-in network in the workplace. Building an expert advisory team is an essential step for the entrepreneur to navigate the complexities of the business world during start-up and throughout the life of the business. The intrapreneur also needs to develop a team to help flesh out the plan and to take the innovation to fruition. Review the questions in Figure 9-2 as you consider the resources that you need to help you move your enterprise forward.

| Questions to Ask | Resources Needed | Support |
|---|---|---|
| Do you have a mentor? | Individual with:<br>• Knowledge of your business<br>• Knowledge skills and experience that you need | • Encourages you in the start-up<br>• Assists with challenges of a new business<br>• Opens doors<br>• Helps you to access resources |
| What type of professional network have you built? | Established network before you get started:<br>• Trusted colleagues<br>• Professional contacts<br>• Community contacts | • People with whom to test out new ideas and explore opportunities<br>• Primary source of business in start-up |
| What type of business advice do you need? | • Lawyer—someone who understands your business<br>• Accountant<br>• Insurance agent<br>• Possibly a personal board of directors or advisory committee | • Saves time and energy<br>• Contracts and legal issues<br>• Financial management, dealing with lenders, accounting<br>• Risk management<br>• Consultation and business advice as needed |

*Continued*

Figure **9-2.** Resources needed by entrepreneurs.

| Questions to Ask | Resources Needed | Support |
|---|---|---|
| How much money do you need to get started? | • Sound business plan<br>• Financial advice | • Accurately assess needs<br>• Communicate and sell your idea to lenders |
| What type of financial reserves do you have available? | • Three to six months' income reserve recommended<br>• Pay off personal debt if possible<br>• Establish personal budget<br>• Money management skills to cope with uneven cash flow | • Support you while your business gets established<br>• Usually takes at least 2 years to achieve a steady revenue |
| What type of support do you have from family and friends? | • Need family and friends on your side<br>• Need their understanding of time and energy required and lifestyle changes | • Source of emotional support<br>• Provide needed advice<br>• Help you to access resources<br>• Help you to market your ideas |

Figure **9-2**, cont'd For legend, see p. 127.

## Reality Check

Once you have gone through your self-assessment, it is time to validate your results with others. Go to trusted colleagues, supervisors, family members, and business advisors to validate your ideas, strengths, and weaknesses. Once you do this, it is time to compare your skills and abilities with the opportunities that you have identified in your scan of the environment. Is there a match? You may work back and forth between these two phases a few times until you can articulate your innovation or business idea a little more clearly. Once you have crystallized the idea and feel confident that it fits your skills and passion, it is time to create a vision for your enterprise or for your innovation within your organization (which we refer to as an "intraprise") (Manion, 1990).

## CREATING THE VISION FOR YOUR ENTERPRISE

"Vision is the stuff of our dreams. Passion is our energy to make it real. The two go together like a horse and rider. In the mind of one is the goal. In the power of the other lies the means to get there" (Bender, 1997, p. 87). Vision and the visioning process are important in the development of an enterprise or intraprise. What is the vision for the business or innovation that you are proposing? A vision helps us to create our reality. Putting it in the form of a statement acts like a strong magnet pulling us toward that possibility (Bopp et al., 1989). Purpose and vision are closely linked. *Purpose* is what you do and why; *vision* is where you are going. Together they are two of the foundational elements that are essential in creating a successful enterprise.

The purpose of a business is expressed as a mission statement that broadly defines the scope of the operation and what distinguishes it from similar businesses (Daft & Fitzgerald, 1992). Take some time to write a purpose or mission statement for your enterprise. This is a creative and important exercise to help you gain clarity about who you are and what you do. The mission statement helps you to communicate your purpose to potential customers, suppliers, and stakeholders. It also helps you to focus your activities on those that support your core purpose.

> The purpose of Connie's business is "to promote paediatric wellness by developing tools and strategies for families to help them care for their children." The purpose of the nurse educators' intraprise is "to promote excellent care to seniors by providing high quality education, mentorship, and consultation to long-term care facilities."

Once you have clarified your purpose, write a vision statement. Imagine what your preferred future is for your enterprise. A vision asks us to stretch and grow; do not be afraid to think big. Once we put our dreams in writing, we start to mobilize all of the forces that help this dream come to life. Review examples of other people's visions that have been successful, and check them against your vision (Bender, 1997). As you go through the process, write down the action steps that will help you achieve the vision. These will become part of your business plan:

> The vision for Connie's business is: "All children are supported by knowledgeable caregivers." The nurse educators' vision statement is: "Care providers in all long-term care facilities have the knowledge and skills to meet the complex needs of their residents."

Check back to your environmental scan and self-assessment. If there is congruence with your purpose and vision, it is time to start putting wheels under the idea with a business plan.

## DEVELOPING YOUR BUSINESS PLAN

*Good things happen by chance. Great things happen when good things are planned.*
**Rosita Hall**

### Why Develop a Business Plan?

Developing a business plan is the equivalent to developing a strategic career plan. A business plan is a more comprehensive document that helps you to tell the story of your proposed enterprise. This is where you put pen to paper to document all of the work and thinking you have done in previous phases. Although business plans have traditionally been linked with developing a new business, they should be developed when considering any new idea, unit, or service. The business plan helps you document all of the relevant facts and ideas about your proposed enterprise in one place, including an organized overview of what you are trying to achieve, why you are trying to achieve it, what it will cost, and the benefits. The business plan is important because it demonstrates the validity of your idea; it will be your primary sales and evaluation tool. It helps you to reflect on the work done to date and helps you to identify gaps and learning needs. Finally, it is a tool to develop business planning and writing skills. A sound business plan is essential to obtaining financing from a lender or to have a project funded. It is important to remember that the business plan is a reflection of you and your ideas. You may want to enlist help from an expert if business writing is not one of your gifts (Manion, 1990). Packaging the plan is also a critical sales feature. It should flow well, look professional, be typed on high-quality paper, and be bound if possible.

### Elements of a Business Plan

The content, length, and complexity of the business plan depend on the purpose and target audience. For example, if the business plan is intended for lenders, the financial elements of the plan should be emphasized. If the plan is detailing an improvement opportunity, the focus should be on the benchmarks and expected outcomes. Organizations often have their own guidelines for writing business plans. The overall goal is to keep it as short as possible while telling the reader the entire story. Writing a good business plan takes effort, but it is well worth the investment. Having a formal plan enables you to respond to changes in the environment and to quickly take advantage of other opportunities as they arise.

A sample outline for a business plan is highlighted in Figure 9-3.

## BRINGING YOUR IDEA TO LIFE: MARKETING AND IMPLEMENTATION

Marketing is the most difficult task for both entrepreneurs and intrapreneurs. It is a conscious and planned activity that requires us to apply our skills in

---

1. **Introduction**
   Summary overview of the proposed idea
2. **Description of the idea, product, or service**
   Fully explains the enterprise: why there is a need, how it works or functions, goals and benefits, comparison to competitors
3. **Organization fit**
   Fit between enterprise and organization; relevance to mission, values, and vision
4. **Market research and analysis**
   Current state; customers; size of market; trends and demographics; potential market penetration; analysis of strengths, weaknesses, opportunities, and threats
5. **Operations plan**
   Organizational structure; people, resources, and equipment needed; location; facilities; hours of operation; operating procedures/standards
6. **Marketing and distribution plan**
   Marketing goals, objectives, and strategies; who will do it; resources required; pricing
7. **Summary of risks**
   Possible risks and impact of products or services; risk management
8. **Development and implementation schedule**
   Implementation tasks, milestones, time frames, responsibilities
9. **Financial plan**
   Budget: revenue, expense, capital costs; financial statements (e.g., balance sheet)
10. **Executive summary**
    Overview of entire plan; hook to catch people to read; written last but positioned first

---

Figure **9-3.** Elements of a business plan. *(Modified from Manion, J. [1990]. Change from within: Nurse intrapreneurs as health care innovators. Chicago: American Nurses Association.)*

new ways. It is really about exchange—a process by which we exchange something of value for something we need (Stern, 1994). The product or service that many nurse entrepreneurs are promoting is their knowledge, skills, and image; they are really marketing themselves (Czaplewski, 1999).

## Marketing Strategies

Stern (1994) uses the "six *Ps*" of marketing as a framework: product, publics, price, place, production, and promotion. *Product* is the service you plan to offer. *Publics* are the people you will serve. *Price* refers to having the right price. *Place* means the location of the service and accessibility by the target market. *Production* is the ability to effectively meet demand. *Promotion* refers to what will motivate people to access your service. The promotion plan is the way you communicate to the public to create an image and motivate people to respond. It includes two elements: your business image and the message (Stern, 1994). Your image, message, mission, values, and target audience will determine the promotion techniques and strategies you will use. Promotion strategies are the methods and tools used to communicate your image and message to the public.

> For Connie the focus of her marketing strategies was in advertising her services and recruiting staff. The nurse educators, on the other hand, realized that they needed not only to market their idea inside the organization to get "buy in," but also to market their idea to the long-term care facilities.

### Communicating Your Business Image

An effective image captures what you want to say to the public, your unique contributions, and what places you apart from others. Everything you do and all materials that you develop communicate image. It is important to remember that a positive image develops over time, whereas a negative image develops quickly and is hard to change. Your image is communicated by your business name; the professionalism and design of all printed and promotional materials, business cards, and letterhead stationery; the language used; the appearance and conduct of everyone who represents you or your business venture; how you talk about competitors; the vehicle you drive; the location, appearance, amenities, and ambiance of your office; communication by telephone; pricing of service; policies for credit; and the actual service that you provide. It is often the small details that make a big impact.

### Promotion Techniques

An effective message engages people to take action and helps them to understand the benefits of doing so. There are numerous techniques for conveying your message. Even though this is the information age, the importance of personal contact and relationships with everyone associated with your venture cannot be underestimated (Schneider, 1997; Stern, 1994).

Networking and mentorship are important promotion strategies. Many communities have small business networking and support groups sponsored by local chambers of commerce or independent business associations. Customer service is imperative to the success of a business or innovation. If you focus on exceeding expectations and then do so, you will never be out of work. Much new business comes from referral by satisfied customers.

Business cards and letterhead stationary are effective and relatively inexpensive promotion tools. Ensure congruence with all printed promotional materials by coordinating your colours, logo, and print on everything, including envelopes, brochures, and proposals. Having access to the Internet, including e-mail has become an essential business tool for marketing, research, and promotion. You may want to consider a website for marketing your services to reach a broad audience and to enable potential clients to have easy access to readily updated information. Speaking at conferences, writing articles in journals, writing letters to the editor, and participating in or sponsoring special events will help to promote your service and develop your profile. Other promotion techniques, including advertising, annual reports, newsletters, direct mail, telemarketing, cold calls, and trade fairs, may all be included in your promotional tool kit depending on your budget, service, and audience.

Marketing requires a sustained effort to produce results and is a continuous process throughout the life of a project or enterprise. You can never afford to let up, even if you are enjoying good fortune. Once you implement the plan, you must evaluate its success and revisit the goals. That brings you back to the start of the career planning cycle.

## JUST DO IT!

Congratulations! You have completed a comprehensive planning process and are now ready to get started. The only way to launch is just to do it. Start telling people about your idea, building your team, and finding your office location—whatever you need to do to get started. Your business plan is your road map. Fear of failure is a great hurdle, but failures often lead to the greatest learning and future innovations. Fear of success is a corollary to fear of failure. Sometimes our success breeds more success and spin-off innovations that challenge our confidence. Are you able to handle the challenges? Without a doubt! Each problem or challenge you overcome along the way prepares you for the next.

## CONCLUSION

Although styles differ, everyone is an innovator and a creator. Every nurse has the ability to be an entrepreneur or intrapreneur. It takes courage, but it is worth the risk. Most entrepreneurs and intrapreneurs have no regrets, and they cite professional, personal, and financial rewards beyond imagination. By integrating ongoing career planning into your professional practice as a continuous process, you will develop the knowledge, skills, and experience that will enable you to seize opportunities that arise.

Danaan Parry (1991) offered this insight about the courage to take risks: "We cast off from the first trapeze in certain faith that we shall catch the one that is flying towards us unseen. If the trapeze is not there, then you might just have the amazing privilege of experiencing the power of flight."

## REFERENCES

Alward, R.R., & Canuñas, C. (1991). *The nurse's guide to marketing*. Florence, KY: Delmar.
Bender, P.U. (1997). *Leadership from within*. Toronto, Ontario, Canada: Stoddart.
Bopp, J. et al. (1989). *The sacred tree*. Twin Lakes: Lotus Light Productions.
Daft, R.L., & Fitzgerald, P.A. (1992). *Management*. Toronto, Ontario, Canada: Dryden Canada.
Czaplewski, L. (1999). Marketing your expertise. *Journal of Intravenous Nursing, 22*(2), 75-80.
Manion, J. (1990). *Change from within. Nurse intrapreneurs as health care innovators.* Chicago: American Nurses Association.
Manion, J. (2001). Enhancing career marketability through intrapreneurship. *Nursing Administration Quarterly, 25*(2), 5-10.
Orga, J. (1996). Becoming a nurse entrepreneur. *Tennessee Nurse, 59*(2), 13-14.
Ortberg, J. (2001). *If you want to walk on water, you've got to get out of the boat*. Grand Rapids, MI: Zondervan.
Parker, M. (1998). The new entrepreneurial foundation for the nurse executive. *Nursing Administration Quarterly, 22*(2), 13-21.
Parry, D. (1991). *Warriors of the heart. A handbook for conflict resolution*. Bainbridge Island, WA: The Earthstewards Network.
Pinchot, G. (1986). *Intrapreneuring: Why you don't have to leave the corporation to become an entrepreneur*. New York: Harper Collins.
Porter-O'Grady, T. (1997). The private practice of nursing: The gift of entrepreneurialism. *Nursing Administration Quarterly, 22*(1), 23-29.
Schneider, B. (1997). Have you thought of entering business as an entrepreneur or intrapreneur, a satisfying alternative career in nursing? *Washington Nurse, 27*(2), 45.
Stern, G.J. (1994). *Marketing workbook for non-profit organizations*. St. Paul, MN: Amherst H. Wilder Foundation.
White, K.R., & Begun, J.W. (1998). Nursing entrepreneurship in an era of chaos and complexity. *Nursing Administration Quarterly, 22*(2), 40-47.

## FURTHER READING

Bygrave, W.D., & Bygrave, B. (1997). *The portable MBS in entrepreneurship* (2nd ed.). New York: John Wiley & Sons.
International Council of Nurses. (1999). *Guidebook for nurse futurists*. Geneva, Switzerland: Author.
Kishel, G.F., & Kishel, P.G. (1996). *How to start and run a successful consulting business*. New York: John Wiley & Sons.
Moore, D.P. (2000). *Careerpreneurs: Lessons from leading women entrepreneurs on building a career without boundaries*. Palo Alto, CA: Davies-Black Publishing.
Norwood, S.L. (1997). *Nurses as consultants: Concepts and processes*. Boston: Addison-Wesley.
Thackray, R. (2002). *20/20 hindsight: From starting up to successful entrepreneur by those who've been there*. London: Virgin Books.
Vallano, A. (1999). *Careers in nursing: Manage your future in the changing world of health care*. New York: Kaplan Books.
Vogel, G., & Doleysh, N. (1994). *Entrepreneuring: A nurse's guide to starting a business*. New York: National League for Nursing.

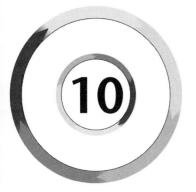

# Planning for Retirement

Margot Young, MA, CHRP

**Margot Young** is President of Margot Young & Associates Ltd. Since 1989 Margot and her associates have provided services in retirement planning, career management, coaching, and creative learning and development programs for organizations. Margot coaches individuals through life and career transitions and takes a special interest in inspiring individuals to grow and develop to their full potential.

## Author Reflections

*As I look ahead to retirement, I realize how exciting it will be to create a retirement as fulfilling as my work life. I now see retirement as a stage in my career, rather than an end. By following the same career planning model I've used throughout my career, I'm confident I can create my ideal retirement!*

*You are old when regrets take the place of dreams.*

*Jimmy Carter*

The world of retirement has changed! If you are one of the thousands of nurses ending your career in the next 10 years or more, your retirement will contrast sharply with the retirement experience of previous generations. In 1975 most nurses worked to age 65 and then looked forward to a quieter, slower lifestyle. Today, however, nurses are retiring earlier, living longer, and participating in a wide range of activities that keep them active, involved, and interested.

There are more opportunities and challenges for nurses nearing retirement than ever before. Just as you have planned the other stages of your career, planning for your retirement will help you take advantage of the many opportunities plus ensure your well-being and security throughout this exciting phase of life. The conditions of your retirement are not preordained; you can have plenty of input about your retirement outcomes *if* you plan ahead.

Ideally you have been planning for retirement since the outset of your career. However, if you are nearing retirement and have not yet started your planning, don't worry. It isn't too late to begin now.

In this chapter you will learn how to apply the Donner-Wheeler Model to your retirement planning. You have many choices to make as you approach retirement. To choose wisely, you must know yourself, your options, and your environment. There may be others to consider besides yourself—spouse, family, relatives, and friends—but you are the one who will need to live with yourself for the next several years. To help you begin the retirement planning process, this chapter focuses on a number of key retirement issues, including health and wellness, housing choices, social needs, finances, working after retirement, and volunteering.

## RETIREMENT AS A WOMEN'S ISSUE

Because nursing is predominantly a female occupation, gender issues arise in relation to retirement. Men and women, who have been socialized differently in the past, have differing attitudes toward money and work. Thomas Yaccato (1996) found that men work for money and power and that work is a major focus of their lives. Although money and power are also important to women, they may rank these lower in relation to other items such as independence, service to others, liking their work, and peer recognition. However, women's roles and attitudes have also changed over the years, and they can no longer be considered a homogeneous group. Younger women's values often differ from those of older women in relation to work, money, and finances. Some women may have mothers who have never worked outside the home and have never had their own money or chequebook; for younger women, this seems almost unbelievable. Today's population of nurses is equally diverse with respect to age-groups and values. At one time most women had to choose between marriage and a career. Now that choice is not necessary, and the majority of nurses successfully combine marriage with a career. Influenced by the women's movement, nurses have become increasingly career oriented, and many have returned to further their education and enhance their career options.

The career decisions that women make can have a strong influence on their future financial security. Traditionally women have been low income earners. This was also true of nurses until quite recently when, with unionization, salaries became more respectable. During their childbearing years, women often move into and out of the workforce and may engage in part-time rather than full-time work. As a result, many women do not have long consecutive years of employment, which affects their pension and other retirement savings plans, as well as their ability to save. Today women have a longer life expectancy than men, and most can expect to outlive their spouse. Yet some married women may believe they will be looked after by their spouse after retirement and therefore do not engage in planning on their own, or they may not even have knowledge of their spouse's retirement plans and financial situation. Those with families may be more interested in paying off the mortgage and saving for the education of their children. Consequently, they may put concerns about pension plans and retirement savings "on the back burner." Although many women, and nurses, continue to develop more independence and financial savvy, others may still be guided by traditional values regarding money and finances.

## THE RETIREMENT PLANNING PROCESS

### Scanning Your Retirement World

In Chapter 2 you learned the importance of scanning your environment and acquired the tools to conduct a scan throughout your career. In planning for retirement, you have some new targets to add to your scanning. You need to keep in touch with what is happening in areas such as health care, pensions, tax changes, housing options, and leisure. Read widely for information regarding legislation and other possible changes that might affect you. Contact the relevant government organizations for updates and information at least 2 years before your retirement. Maintain contact with a financial planner or your bank manager, read the various financial institution newsletters, and obtain annual updates on proposed or debated changes, as well as actual changes relevant to your own situation. Your professional organizations may also have useful information to help you keep abreast of changes that could affect your retirement.

If you are employed in an organization, learn about the various options for retirement from the human resources department and/or your union. You may not be aware of certain early retirement options. Learn all the details, and find out what it would give you in actual income. And of course, use your network! Speak to recently retired friends and colleagues who have been through the array of information, red tape, and regulations, and learn from their experiences. This is also a good time to look at your professional nursing organization to determine what support, benefits, and help it may be able to provide as you plan your retirement. The box on p. 138 is a beginning scan of current retirement trends; this will provide you with a context in which to conduct your environmental scan.

### Assessing Yourself: Creating the Foundation for Planning

Just as conducting a regular self-assessment was an important part of your career planning strategy, it also is the cornerstone of a successful retirement. In Chapter 3 you learned the importance of knowing yourself and your interests, values, and skills. As you prepare for retirement, it is important to revisit what you have learned about yourself and to use this information in creating your vision and your plan for retirement. The following sections present some key aspects of self to consider.

#### What Do You Get from Your Work?

People who identify strongly with their career often experience a loss of identity when they retire. Work provides many intangible benefits and fills many needs as well as supplying a paycheque. This is especially true for nurses

---

### Retirement Trends Today

1. People are retiring at a younger age and are healthier than in the past. In general, the average age of retirees in the developed world ranges from 58 to 62 years of age (Jackson, 2002).
2. Income and economic levels among retirees has risen (Jackson, 2002).
3. Retirees are more active and involved in the community and world.
4. More people than ever before engage in some form of work after retirement. In 1997, 40% of retirees in Canada between 55 and 59 years of age returned to work (Statistics Canada, 2002). A recent survey indicated that 80% plan to engage in some form of work after retirement (American Association of Retired Persons, 1999).
5. Housing and home options are increasing. These range from moving to a cottage, country property, or mobile home; downsizing from a house to a condo; home-sharing; and more.
6. The population is aging. By 2030, one in every four people in the developed world will be at least 50 years of age. By 2050, 50% of continental Europe will be at least 49 years of age (Jackson, 2002).
7. Some governments are reducing their level of financial support for retirees or are considering an increase in the age at which government pension benefits begin. Other governments are encouraging individuals and organizations to contribute a greater share of retirement income (Jackson, 2002).
8. There will be much greater usage of national health care systems as the population ages around the globe (Jackson, 2002).

---

whose work is critical to the health and well-being of others and whose motivation is so often tied to the need and wish to make a difference to people. The practice of nursing brings the additional benefits of social contacts and support and being involved in important decisions. Before you make any decisions about retirement, ask yourself, "What does work give me? What are the specific rewards work has provided for me, and how important are these rewards for me?"

Once you have made the decision to retire, it is time to start determining what your retirement will look like.

### What Are Your Priorities?

As you approach retirement, you might discover that your priorities have changed. Life circumstances can trigger a reshuffling of priorities. For example, if you have devoted your life to the care of others, including family members, you might want to give more time to yourself in retirement to satisfy your personal goals and interests. Or, conversely, retirement may provide you with the opportunity to spend more time with family or friends who need help and support. Consider writing out your top five priorities for retirement.

If you are living with a partner, encourage him or her to do the same exercise. Then share your lists and brainstorm how both of you can incorporate your priorities into your retirement vision and plan.

### What Are Your Skills and Talents?

Now it is time to decide which of the many skills you have developed over the years will be valuable to you in your retirement, whether for personal use, volunteer work, or paid work. You may want to use or develop totally different skills, or you may want to use your current skills in a completely different environment. As an active nurse you have spent your career helping and caring; as a retired nurse you may want to continue using your helping skills in your community.

> Leon, a nurse manager, enjoyed coordinating projects and people. He enjoyed being the leader in projects and realized that he was gifted in pulling together resources and people and in getting projects off the ground. Leon plans to continue using his skills in coordinating and working with people and will look into serving on the board of an organization he was connected with as part of his job. Completing a thorough self-assessment before he started his retirement planning helped Leon identify a retirement direction.

### What is Your Desired Financial Picture?

You have had to consider your financial situation in planning each step of your career, whether when returning to school, considering a career change, or deciding when to take time out to start a family. Financial planning takes on even more importance as you plan for retirement. You will need to assess your current financial situation and how much money you will need to live your desired lifestyle. A number of good financial planning books with spreadsheet exercises can help you determine your income and expenses currently, as well as your projected income and expenses in retirement. You cannot fully determine your financial needs until you have created your vision for retirement.

You also need to know how much pension income you might receive from employer pensions (if you are enrolled in one) and from government sources. In general, these sources provide only partial income, and you are expected to provide a percentage of your retirement income from your own savings. The amount of retirement income an individual is expected to provide varies from country to country. Your environmental scanning will show you how much you need to save for your retirement.

As you approach retirement, you will need to take specific action to activate retirement income from your organization and from government sources. Begin to investigate these action steps at least 2 years before your planned retirement. You might want to consider the possibility of working with a financial planner to help you put together your financial picture. If so, be sure to get references from people you trust, and ensure that the individual you select is accredited and experienced.

### Are You Ready to Retire?

Answering this question is not easy. Completing the self-assessment in Chapter 3 and reflecting on the previous questions will have given you a clearer picture of your current needs, interests, and values. Reflecting on the questions in the previous section will help you determine if this is the right time for you to retire. Are most of your needs being met through work? Would more of your needs be met if you retired? Some nurses who want to retire but who lack the necessary funds retire from their nursing position and find or create a job that provides sufficient income for retirement and addresses their retirement needs, interests, and values.

People are increasingly considering early retirement. You may see many of your colleagues retire before you and wish to be in their situation. You could conceivably live for another 25 to 30 years after early retirement; such freedom may sound appealing initially but may pall after a few years. Many people actively embrace this choice for the freedom it gives them to pursue other interests in the later stages of their lives. Ideally, the process of deciding whether early retirement is the right option for you should be the same as the one you use for regular retirement planning. That is, it should be based on the same type of self-assessment to determine your needs and choices as if you opted to retire at the more usual age of 60 or 65.

You may, as part of your assessment, decide that you need to build in a transition period before your full retirement. In this case, you may consider part-time work, even outside of nursing, or consulting or teaching in your area of expertise as a means of easing into retirement. The volunteer work you select at this stage of your retirement may especially help you fulfill your needs and gradually put the elements of your new lifestyle in place.

> Marie, who is 54 years old, and her husband, who is 10 years older, decided they both would retire at the same time. When Marie's hospital offered early retirement packages, she accepted. After 3 years of retired life, however, Marie was restless. She missed the interaction with patients and other nurses. She discussed the situation with her husband and realized that she needed some focus outside her home. She subsequently found volunteer work with palliative care patients for the local health department. Spending time with patients and attending meetings of the palliative care team fulfilled Marie's need for patient and peer contact and provided inner satisfaction.

The lesson here is that if you are continuously engaged in career planning and development and know who you are and what you like and want, you will already have planned a suitable lifestyle when it is time to retire.

## Your Retirement Vision

Do you have a dream that has been patiently waiting in the back of your mind while you fulfilled life's obligations? Or perhaps you have a dream you have forgotten all about? Now is the time to bring those dreams forward and give them space to grow. You can do that by letting them materialize in your mind, by discussing them with others, and by imagining how you might begin to realize those dreams. Perhaps for the first time in your life you can structure your time in a way that meets your needs.

One of the joys of retirement is that you can experiment with new things without the concerns you had when you were building your career. For example, in a paid career role you might be concerned about moving to another job or speaking out about something you don't agree with for fear of hurting your career or working relationships. In retirement, if you don't like something—whether it is a new part-time job, volunteer work, or a club you have joined—you can simply change your course and move on to something different. This is a new mindset, and it takes time to become accustomed to it. Once you do, however, you will be pleased at how liberating that thought is. As you create your vision, there are many aspects of retirement to consider.

### Leisure

In retirement you have the luxury of time to focus on your favourite activities and explore new ones. If you have given most of your time and energy to career or family, you may need to develop some new interests. Childhood interests and activities often provide clues regarding pursuits that might hold your interest and passion in retirement.

Consider the full range of leisure activities—hobbies, sports, clubs, cultural activities, music, entertaining, learning and self-development, volunteer work, community work, spiritual, travel, and creative pursuits such as painting or writing. Consider selecting at least one, if not more, hobby or interest to incorporate into your retirement plan.

### Friends and Relationships

As you leave your professional work world behind, you have a wonderful opportunity to consider who you would like to have as part of your new support network. If most of your social contacts are with work colleagues, now is the time to consider developing new friendships. Can you rekindle lost or forgotten friendships from the past? Places to meet people with similar interests and values include volunteer work, alumni associations, professional organizations, community or faith groups, and sports or hobby groups. With so many people reaching retirement age at the same time, there's an excellent chance that others like you will be interested in making new friends to share times together.

> Theresa thrived on the daily contacts she had in her nursing career. She continues meeting people and making new friends through her work on a community agency board, by getting involved with a woman's network, and by playing tennis regularly.

Of course, you won't want to ignore the many friends you made through your worklife, and retirement is an opportunity to enrich those long-term relationships. Professional organizations often provide the perfect "meeting place" for keeping those relationships going.

If you have a partner, is that partner also retiring, and have you shared your vision for retirement? Couples face unique challenges in retirement. Although the opportunity to spend more time together can be welcoming, it also presents challenges. You might discover that you and your partner have different interests and goals for your retirement years. For example, your partner may have a greater need for quiet, alone time, but you may picture spending more time together or with family and friends. The best way to retire harmoniously with your partner is to share your personal vision and encourage your partner to develop his or her own vision. Then discuss your visions together and work out a plan that accommodates both. Usually some compromise and a good sense of humour are required!

### *Living a Healthy Retirement*

Although many nurses counsel others on strategies to maintain or acquire optimum levels of wellness, they may not take their own advice. Now is the time to practice all those good habits you encourage others to follow! If you don't currently follow a fitness program, make this a part of your retirement plan. A regular program tailored to your own health needs will give you improved health and enhanced emotional and psychological well-being.

Your mental and emotional health affects your physical health, your enjoyment of life, and your ability to deal with life's ups and downs. Thoughts become habitual over time. By focusing on the positive in a situation and on what you can control in life, you promote your own well-being and health. Consider physical and mental fitness an important part of your retirement plan. Now is the time to take all the good advice you have been giving clients over the years and act on it yourself.

### *Where Do You Want to Live?*

In retirement, you have the freedom to choose where you want to live. The number of options for housing and lifestyle choices is unlimited and will continue expanding to meet the requirements of the baby boomers.

Before moving to a new residence or location, ask yourself the questions listed in the box below, and discuss them with others involved in the move.

---

#### Questions to Consider Before You Move

1. What are my priorities and values? Do I want to live near family and friends, or is it more important to live in an area that supports my interests?
2. Will this move/new home accommodate any potential physical limitations for the next 10, 20, or 30 years?
3. How well do I know the area to which I'm planning to relocate? Research well before making any move. If considering a move, plan at least one long trip to "test out" living in the new location. If feasible, lease your apartment or home for a year or 6 months rather than sell.

Living alone as one grows older is a concern for many. Communities are being built in which groups of like-minded individuals live in their own homes yet share common facilities. Aging-in-place facilities are becoming more common as well; in such facilities people can move from their own apartment or house onto a floor where care is provided. Your environment scanning will help you become aware of what is available in your area.

### Working After Retirement

More retired people are choosing to continue working beyond retirement. Many nurses are retiring earlier, and do not feel ready to completely leave the workforce. Others continue working for financial reasons. As the population ages and requires more health care, retired nurses will have a wealth of work possibilities in many areas. Opportunities for self-employment or for part-time, full-time, or contract work exist in both traditional and non-traditional health care areas. Some people prefer to work in totally new areas. To help you sort through the possibilities, it is useful to ask yourself the questions listed in the box below.

### Should I Work After Retirement?

1. What is my goal in working: To use my expertise? To earn a substantial amount of money? To stay connected with people? To help others?
2. Do I want to remain in health care or try something different?
3. How much time do I want to work? A few hours a week? Evenings? Days? Only in the cold weather? For short periods of time?
4. What are some areas of interest I could work in? What are some of my dreams about post-retirement worklife?

### Volunteering

Volunteer work provides structure, meaning, and a way to meet others. It also is a way to develop new skills and interests and is a wonderful way to give back to the community. Most cities and towns have volunteer centres that match people with volunteer opportunities. Your nursing network is also a terrific source of potential volunteer activities. The range of possibilities is enormous—from reading to a small child in school, to mentoring a new graduate for an hour each week, to volunteering in a long-term care setting. Just as you reviewed your interests, skills, and values before considering your next career move, use this same process to find the right volunteer role for you. Now you are ready to create your retirement plan.

## Your Retirement Plan

The strategies you learned in Chapter 5 to develop a career plan also apply when planning your retirement. To keep your plan alive and help it grow, discuss it with family and friends. As previously mentioned, your partner or others who are part of your plan need to be fully involved at all stages. Keep in mind, however, that it is important to live fully today while planning for tomorrow.

It is important to inject a good dose of reality into your planning. What are the restraining factors that might challenge you in meeting your retirement goals? View them not as roadblocks, but merely as obstacles or hurdles. With persistence, trust, and creative problem solving you might find a way around your obstacles so that you adjust, not give up, your priorities and dreams.

Retirement, although an exciting time of life for most nurses today, is also a major life change. Think back to the self-assessment you completed in Chapter 3 and reflect on how you have managed other major changes in your life. The strategies you have used in the past to cope with change—at work as well as in your personal life—will help you deal with your transition to retirement. If there is anything at which nurses are experts, it is managing change. William Bridges (1991) says that transition can be a wonderful time of exploration, creativity, and growth. He reinforces the importance of finding interests or pursuits to replace the inevitable losses that change brings. Include in your plan interests or pursuits that will replace any potential losses you might experience in retirement.

Many retired nurses say they are so busy they do not know how they ever had time to work. Retired people find that expectations and demands on their time from family, community, and volunteer groups can increase once they leave their job. Create a balanced retirement by including in your plan goals based on your priorities and interests in four areas: physical, social, emotional, and financial. Then market your plan. Communicate your goals to others in your life so they know your plans.

## CONCLUSION

In this chapter we explained how to use the Donner-Wheeler Model to plan your retirement. In retirement you will continue to change, and so will the environment around you. If your retirement no longer is satisfying and fulfilling, you now have the skills and knowledge to review and adjust your plan. With planning, a positive approach, and a willingness to learn and explore, you can create the retirement you want.

This final phase of your career is a time for you to explore and fulfill your interests and dreams and to grow in new and different ways. After many years of hard work in your chosen profession, you deserve a great retirement. Enjoy the journey!

## REFERENCES

Bridges, W. (1991). *Transitions: Making sense of life's changes*. Reading, MA: Addison-Wesley.
Jackson, R. (2002). *The global retirement crisis*. Washington, DC: The Center for Strategic and International Studies.

Roper Starch Worldwide. (1999). *Baby boomers envision their retirement: An AARP segmentation analysis*. Washington, DC: AARP.

Statistics Canada. (2002). Approaching Retirement (September 26). *The Daily*.

Yaccato, T. (1996). *Balancing act: A Canadian woman's financial success guide* (rev. ed.) Scarborough, Ontario, Canada: Prentice-Hall.

## FURTHER READING

Autry, J. (2002). *The spirit of retirement: Creating a life of meaning and personal growth*. Roseville, CA: Prima Publications.

Bond, D., & Bond, D. (2002). *Future perfect: Retirement strategies for productive people*. Vancouver, British Columbia, Canada: Douglas & McIntyre.

Bronfman, E. (2002). *The third act: Reinventing yourself after retirement*. New York: G.P. Putman's Sons.

Chapman, E. (1997). *Comfort zones*, Menlo Park, CA: Crisp Publications.

Critchley, R. (2002). *Rewired, rehired, or retired: A global guide for the experienced worker*. San Francisco: John Wiley & Sons.

Nelson, M. (1998). *Strong women stay young*. New York: Bantam Books.

Vaillant, G. (2002). *Aging well: Surprising guideposts to a happier life from the landmark Harvard Study of Adult Development*. Boston: Little, Brown.

Waitley, D., & Sayfer, E. (1995). *How to be happily retired*. Berkeley, CA: Celestial Arts.

# PART III

# Career Planning and Development in the Future

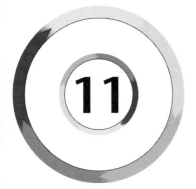

### Chapter Eleven

# Organizational Career Development: A Priority for the Future

Gail J. Donner, RN, PhD and Mary M. Wheeler, RN, MEd

▰ Author Reflections

*If we have learned one thing over the course of our work, it is that to sustain nursing for the future, we need to build cultures in workplaces where nurses can talk about their careers, not just their jobs, and where employers see supporting nursing careers as a benefit for themselves as well as for their employees.*

*Never leave well enough alone.*

*Loewy*

As we write this book, the world and the workplace are facing turbulent times. We know that from these times of change will emerge new opportunities, new ways of doing things, and new perspectives, but the journey will certainly have its share of bumps along the way. As we embrace the future, it is important to consider the challenges ahead. In this chapter, we discuss how career planning and development, embedded in an organization's strategic plan, can be a valuable tool for developing career-resilient employees and why it must be a priority to ensure a healthy future for nursing.

## DEVELOPING A CAREER DEVELOPMENT CULTURE

As we learned in Chapter 2, the health care environment is experiencing a great deal of change and, in the midst of that change, nursing around the world is facing a serious and unprecedented shortage of nurses. Recruitment and retention of nurses is something that employers, educators, policy-makers, and the public are struggling with and will likely continue to consider a priority over the next several decades. It is clear that the world of nursing must change if we are to meet the human resource needs of the future.

The social contract between employers and employees has shifted, "from an expectation of long term to a transitory relationship; from perception of entitlement to shared responsibility; from employees being part of an organization to being a factor in production; and from corporations taking a patriarch's role to employees bearing more of the responsibility" (Altman & Post, 1996, p. 51). The new employees have also changed the paradigm from which they operate and seek employers who are responsive to their learning and professional needs and their particular life stage and who provide them with environments that encourage them to do their best work. To create an environment that meets employees' needs while striving to meet their own objectives, employers must seek to develop a career development culture that encourages continuous lifelong learning and emphasizes and rewards flexibility over the career lifetime of employees. "The responsibility for a person's own career planning must be that of the individual, but the responsibility for the success of a career development culture requires the active support and involvement of three principal actors: top management, supervisors and employees themselves" (Conger, 2002, p. 371). This is a major challenge for both the employer and the employee. The employer needs the flexibility to respond quickly to changing internal and external forces with new and better ways of getting the work done. Employees need to be prepared to explain how their skills make them suitable for a newly created job or role and have the confidence to risk taking on the new work.

The real winners in this new environment will be the organizations that focus on the human side of change and assist their employees to be proactive and to take charge of their careers. The literature is replete with examples of incentives focusing on recruiting and retaining, and many of these strategies have yielded at least short-term results. However, it is only when the culture itself changes and is able to focus on the individual's career resilience that employers will be able to recruit and retain over the long term. One strategy that helps build this culture is the implementation of an integrated comprehensive career development program.

## AN INTEGRATED COMPREHENSIVE CAREER DEVELOPMENT PROGRAM

Organizational career development programs that align employee development planning and organizational strategic planning can be effective for both the organization and the individual. Career development programs, including onsite and online workshops and career coaching for individuals and groups, are resources to assist employees in ongoing learning and self-assessment and allow them to take risks and grow within the changing institution rather than leave it. The inclusion of programs that also develop nurse career coaches *within* the organization assist in building the organization's capacity to sustain a career-resilient nursing workforce. Career-resilient workers are dedicated to the idea of continuous learning, are ready to reinvent themselves to keep pace with change, take responsibility for their own career management, and are committed to the organization's success (Waterman, Waterman, & Collard, 1994).

Thus an organizational career development program fosters the relationship between individual career plans and the organization's needs (Figure 11-1). Employees, managers, and the organization all have necessary and specific roles to play in a career development program. Gutteridge, Leibowitz, and Shore (1993) advise employees to assess themselves and develop career plans compatible with the organizational realities. Managers are encouraged to support their employees and help them to understand the organization's needs and requirements, and the organization is responsible for providing the tools, resources, and structures to support the process.

## The People

The people involved in this career development initiative include the employees being helped to plan their careers so they can meet the changing needs of the workplace (the participants) and those who assist participants with their career planning and development (the providers).

### The Participants: Diverse Populations Require Diverse Solutions

It is absolutely critical that all nurses, regardless of their tenure with the organization or their experience in nursing, be included in any career programming. Just as we customize client care based on a variety of environmental and demographic characteristics, so must we provide career programs to meet the diverse needs of nurses at every stage of the career continuum. This means there must be programs that help new recruits see how their goals can fit with the organization's and that help them learn to navigate the sometimes turbulent waters of the workplace. Workshops and coaching can provide a safe place for new recruits to learn to articulate their career goals, find colleagues who can support and mentor them, and understand the organizational politics and processes. In addition, workshops and coaching help reduce some of the discouragement and disillusionment often felt by new graduates and new employees. New recruits are a vulnerable group in health care organizations. We do not want and cannot afford to lose them, but we will if we do not target them for attention that meets their specific needs.

Mid-career nurses compose another vulnerable population and, as we learned in Chapter 8, their needs are very different. Workshops and coaching provide them with the opportunity to reflect and re-energize, articulate their vision for their future, and see that their desired future is possible within the organization and within nursing. These nurses, who generally do not feel appreciated, could be recognized for their experience and offered enhanced (not additional) roles as mentors, intrapreneurs, consultants, preceptors, and career coaches, to name just a few. In return, the organization is able to retain invaluable resources.

Other groups that require individualized career attention include younger nurses who are coping with young families and need a workplace that is willing to invest in them in the short term to see the return on investment develop in the long term. Older nurses, struggling with less energy and with

**Organizational Needs**

What are the organization's major strategic issues over the next 2 to 3 years?

- What are the most critical needs and challenges that the organization will face over the next 2 to 3 years?
- What critical skills, knowledge, and experience will be needed to meet these challenges?
- What staffing levels will be required?
- Does the organization have the bench strength necessary to meet the critical challenges?

**Issue**

Are employees developing themselves in a way that links personal effectiveness and satisfaction with the achievement of the organization's strategic objectives?

**Individual Career Needs**

How do I find career opportunities within the organization that:

- Use my strengths
- Address my developmental needs
- Provide challenge
- Match my interests
- Match my values
- Match my personal style

Figure **11-1.** Career development systems. Linking organizational needs with individual career needs. *(From Gutteridge, T., Leibowitz, Z., & Shore, J. [1993]. Organizational career development: Benchmarks for building a world-class workforce. San Francisco: Jossey-Bass.)* This material is used by permission of John Wiley & Sons, Inc.

the demands of aging parents or partners, also require help in meeting their career needs while continuing to contribute to the organization's mission and mandate. They require more varied and flexible work. Nurses from diverse cultural and ethnic backgrounds, men, and others who are may be considered "visible minorities" need to have the opportunity to learn how their distinctive career needs can be met within the organization. It is clear we also want to encourage nurses who are considering taking on leadership roles within the organization, and career planning programs must form an important part of organizational succession planning—a strategy to ensure continuity of leadership by developing the talent within.

### The Providers: How Leaders Fit In

Employers who acknowledge that they need to pay attention to employees' career development often do not know where to begin. Some managers agree that they have a role to play in assisting employees with their career planning and development; but they are also trying to cope with the turbulent work environment, are not sure about their own futures, and do not believe they have the skill. If managers are to fulfill a professional development role, it must be clearly identified; its connection to performance appraisal, promotion, and opportunities for change and growth must be articulated; and the manager must be helped to develop the required coaching and mentoring skills. This can be accomplished through courses, workshops, and formal education in human resource management. In addition, the managers themselves need support and mentoring. They need superiors who help them take control of their careers, who take an interest in their potential, who help them identify their strengths and limitations, and who help them plan their growth and development. In other words, they need senior managers who model enlightened human resource management, especially in difficult times.

Donner, Waddell, and Wheeler (1996) reported that, more often than not, nurses in their survey did not seek out their nurse manager for career development advice. In addition, it is clear that managers do not necessarily possess the skills required to assist staff (Donner & Wylie, 1995). As Jeska and Rounds (1996) found when they reviewed various career development programs, significant attention was focused on managers, who were deemed critical to creating an effective environment for career development. The presence of unique, innovative models were believed to be the result of a progressive nurse's leadership.

There are a number of opportunities for managers to assist staff with career planning, including at recruitment, at time of hire, at regular performance appraisals, throughout employment, and at the exit interview (Figure 11-2). Their role as coach, support, and mentor make the difference in staff satisfaction, productivity, and turnover, as well as in their own job satisfaction.

Attending to the career needs of employees is also a role for informal leaders in an organization. Advanced practice nurses, clinical educators, resource

## Recruitment

This is where your career developer role begins. In the initial interview with a prospective employee:

- Become familiar with the candidate's career goals.
- Determine whether and how you can help him or her meet those goals.
- Talk about how your unit/agency fits the candidate's objectives.

## At Time of Hire

Work with the employee to develop short-term and long-term objectives:

- Make the career plan part of the employee record.
- The plan should include not only practice objectives related to patient care but also development objectives (e.g., committee, professional work) and educational goals.

## At Regular Performance Appraisal

- Review objectives, paying attention to professional development and educational objectives.
- Work *together* with the employee to revisit the plan, evaluate progress to date, and determine any revisions/subtractions/additions to the plan.

## Ongoing

- Spend time on a regular basis discussing professional development opportunities.
- Ensure that staff see you as a resource or, if you feel your skills are limited, as access to a resource.
- Make sure staffing plans (daily and long-term) recognize the need for development and allow time for that development.
- Keep informed yourself regarding opportunities in your agency and in the field in general.

## Exit Interview

- When an employee leaves, whether through internal transfer or outside employment, you have an opportunity to review career goals and to obtain feedback on how you have helped the employee's development.

Figure **11-2.** The manager's role in career planning.

nurses, staff nurses, and others can provide coaching support to their colleagues if they are willing and are helped to develop the requisite skills. If programs are created to assist those leaders with interest and potential to develop their career coaching skills, then the organization accomplishes two things. First, it has a cadre of providers who are available to coach staff; this can reduce or eliminate their reliance on outside consultants. Second, they provide an enriched career opportunity for those individuals. It is a win-win situation for both the nurse leaders, who are looking for ways to enhance their own careers, and for the employer, who is building capacity and sustainability within the organization.

Lance Secretan (1999) calls on leaders to help staff find their passion—where their interests and skills intersect with energizing, fulfilling work. The more they can engage individuals in their own self-exploration, the more energy they will have for directing themselves toward work they can master and enjoy.

## The Programs: What Are the Components?

As we have already said, career development programs need to reflect the needs of the participants and the mission of the organization. If a program is to be truly comprehensive, it must be integrated into the organization's values, human resource policies, and processes. It is not just a matter of designing and implementing programs and services; rather it is about supporting them and resourcing them appropriately. To ensure success, an integrated comprehensive organizational career development program requires a champion; a steering committee; well-articulated communication strategies; formalized links with Human Resources, Organizational and Professional Development, and other key departments; and a variety of excellent products customized to the populations to be served—whether they are new recruits, mid-career nurses, managers, or informal leaders. Also required is the need for accessibility and flexibility to ensure the programs offered meet the needs and climate of the organization.

The programs should include career planning and development workshops and coaching that are available both onsite and online. These offerings help nurses understand how to integrate the organization's vision and strategy with their own strengths and goals. Traditionally workshops and coaching have been offered onsite, thus requiring nurses to come to the program or service. In the current climate, with even greater shortages projected for the future, organizations are being forced to decrease opportunities for nurses to leave the bedside to participate in continuing education programs. This trend, along with the increasing number of younger and more technologically savvy nurses and the pressure to recruit and retain more of these nurses, has led to a growing demand for online continuing education. Thus offering career planning and development workshops and coaching both onsite and online is a must. These workshops should provide nurses with an opportunity to review their careers to date, to learn strategies to assist them in making future career decisions, and to identify support systems as they move through the career planning and development process. Ultimately the workshops should provide practical strategies for making career planning an integral part of everyday practice.

Running concurrently to the workshops should be the opportunity for participants to access individual career coaching. Career coaching is a powerful tool to promote career resilience and job satisfaction. It helps staff integrate their vision for their own career futures with the organization's mission and goals.

Becoming a nurse career coach offers a new career path for nurses who are looking for opportunities to develop themselves and support their colleagues. Nurses in formal and informal leadership roles who are provided with opportunities to develop career-coaching competencies can also take an active role in assisting colleagues to achieve their career goals.

For an integrated comprehensive career planning and development program to be successful, the organization needs to provide access not only to workshops and coaching but also to career opportunities. It is not enough for nurses to articulate their career vision if they are unable to see where and how that vision can be realized through opportunities in the organization. An up-to-date inventory of internal resources/career opportunities, jobs online, skills bank inventory, and a resource centre are some of the strategies that need to be in place and accessible to sustain this initiative. In addition to these strategies, staff development initiatives focused on continuous learning, including in-house programs to meet the employee's and the employer's needs, must be made available. These programs need to support the advancement of individual careers and the organization's goals, thereby ensuring that both parties grow and develop. In the same way, clinical educators must ensure that orientation programs, clinical skills programs, and general professional education programs are integrated with the performance management and career development programs that the workplace provides.

## Evaluation and Research: Critical for Success

Implementing an integrated comprehensive career development program into any organization is not easy and requires significant investment of human, material, and financial resources. Therefore it is important that the return on the investment be visible and significant. To ensure that the providers, participants, and payers are satisfied with their initial investment, an evaluation component should be built into the design and implementation of any program. This requires all of the players in the program to articulate their goals and expected outcomes at the outset. Indicators of success for the organization may be reduced turnover, fewer grievances, reduced absenteeism, and other similar measurable outcomes. For both the employer and the employee, increased levels of job satisfaction, more competition for available leadership opportunities, and increased participation in non-required organizational activities may be other desired outcomes.

As with many other professional development initiatives, measuring the "softer" outcomes is complicated and not always precise. We do, however, need to begin somewhere. Just as the career development program must be integrated into the other organizational professional development activities, so must the evaluation and ongoing research be integrated into the organization's quality management programs. Agreement by all the players regarding the outcomes to be measured and the indicators of success is the place to begin. From there, it is a work in progress. What is critical is that we learn from our experience and seek to practice evidence-based professional development programming just as we seek to provide evidence-based patient care.

## CONCLUSION

If a competent and confident workforce is the key to organizational success, then leadership in career development is not an option for employers. Career enhancement programs now appear in many workplaces. If organizations are to be successful, employees must learn how to use the opportunities these programs provide. A career development program provides employees with a framework for asking the questions that enable them to discover opportunities within the workplace and how to capitalize on them. Such programs help employees become responsible for taking action over their own careers and for finding opportunities to achieve their career "visions" within their current workplaces. Employers benefit in return because these newly prepared and career-resilient nurses are able to work "with" them to create the health care delivery system of the future.

Matthews (2001) says that organizations need to evolve to a point where they understand (1) that employees are valuable resources that need to be supported and guided in their career development, and (2) that employees have the freedom to plan and manage their own careers, to access the tools required to do that, and to make their own career choices. In addition, organizations need to create a coaching culture, "a culture that provides employees with unfettered access to support and guidance to develop their careers" (p. 29). That is our challenge for the future.

## REFERENCES

Altman, B.W., & Post, J.E. (1996). Beyond the "social contract": An analysis of the executive view at twenty-five large companies. In D.T. Hall & Associates (Eds.), *The career is dead—Long live the career* (pp. 46-71). San Francisco: Jossey-Bass.

Conger, S. (2002). Fostering a career development culture: Reflections on the roles of managers, employees, and supervisors. *Career Development International, 7*(6), 371-375.

Donner, G., Waddell, J., & Wheeler, M. (1996). *Career planning and development: An evaluation project.* Toronto, Ontario, Canada: Provincial Nursing Administrators Interest Group.

Donner, G., & Wylie, D. (1995). *The nurse manager in Ontario hospitals: The crucial link to quality work environments.* Toronto, Ontario, Canada: Ontario Ministry of Health, Nursing Innovation Program.

Gutteridge, T., Leibowitz, Z., & Shore, J. (1993). *Organizational career development.* San Francisco: Jossey-Bass.

Jeska, S., & Rounds, R. (1996). Addressing the human side of change: Career development and renewal. *Nursing Economics, 14,* 339-345.

Matthews, V. (2001). Coaching career development strategies for competitive advantage: Finding freedom from within. *Career Planning and Adult Development Journal, 17*(1), 27-32.

Secretan, L. (1999). *Inspirational leadership.* Toronto, Ontario, Canada: Macmillan Canada.

Waterman, R.H., Waterman, J.A., & Collard, B.J. (1994). Toward a career-resilient workforce. *Harvard Business Review, 72*(4), 87-95.

## FURTHER READING

Handy, C. (1989). *The age of unreason.* London: Arrow Books.

Hall, D.T. (1986). *Career development in organizations.* San Francisco: Jossey-Bass.

Knowdell, R. (1996). *Building a career development program.* Palo Alto, CA: Davies-Black.

Kummerow, J. (1991). *New directions in career planning and the workplace.* Palo Alto, CA: Davies-Black.

London, M. (1995). *Employees, careers, and job creation.* San Francisco: Jossey-Bass.

# Index

## A

Academic environment
  scanning, 95
  self-marketing in, 99-103
Accomplishments
  feedback regarding, 30
  self-evaluation of, 26f, 28, 97
  of students, 97
Affirmation, 40
Awards, as listed in résumé, 73

## B

Beliefs
  self-evaluation of, 24, 96
  self-limiting, 39
  of students, 96
Business advise, 128f
Business image, communication of,
  132-133
Business plans, 130-131
  elements of, 130-131, 131f
  importance of, 130
Business skills, 125-126

## C

Career changing goals, 46
Career counselors, 31-32
Career development
  control of, 10-11
  organizational. *See*
    Organizational career
    development.
Career goals
  assessment and evaluation
    of, 59
  change in career direction to
    achieve, 48-50
  establishing
    in career action plan, 45-50
    criteria for, 47
  indicators of success of, 48,
    52f-57f, 59
  types of, 46
Career objective, as listed in
  résumé, 73

Career plan
  action plan for, 50-59
  assessment and evaluation
    of, 59
  elements of, 51
  example of, 52f-57f
  development of, 8-9, 44-62
  issues in, 45-59
  resources for, 51-58, 52f-57f,
    58b
  example of, 52f-57f
  indicators of success of, 51,
    52f-57f, 59
  maintaining flexibility in, 59
  start date for, 50-51
Career planning, 4-5, 44-45
  future of, 147-158
  during loss of job, 59-61
  by students, 93-104
Career summary, as listed in
  résumé, 73
Career vision, 35-37
  career options from, 41-42
  creation of, 8, 34-43
  of entrepreneurs/intrepreneurs,
    129-130
  grounding of, 111, 111f, 116-117
  at mid-career, 111, 111f,
    114-115
  of students, 98-99
Chief of nursing practices, 18
Clinical environment, scanning, 95
Clinical placements, 97-98
  interviews for, 102
Community experience, as listed in
  résumé, 77
Community health, 16
Computerization, influences
  of, 15
Consumer-driven models, of
  health care delivery, 15
Counselors, career, 31-32
Cover letters, 78-80
  elements of, 80f
  sample of, 81f
Curriculum vitae (CV), 67, 68f

---

Page numbers followed by *f* refer to figures; page numbers followed by *b* refer to boxes.

161

Organizational career *(Continued)*
  evaluation and research of,
    156-157
  providers in, 153-155

**P**

Patient care executives, 18
Patients, as consumers, 15
Performance appraisals, managers
  and, 154f
Personal qualities, self-assessment
  of, 27, 125-126
Presentations
  listed in résumé, 77
  as self-marketing technique, 87
Priorities
  at mid career, 113f
  in retirement planning, 138-139
Professional memberships and
  affiliations, 77
Promotion techniques, for
  entrepreneurs/intrepreneurs,
    132-133
Provider-driven models, of health
  care delivery, 15
Publication(s)
  listed in résumé, 77
  writing for, 80-82

**R**

Realignment, 50
Reality check, 29-31
  by entrepreneurs/intrepreneurs,
    129
  by students, 98
Recruitment, and employee career
  development, 154f
References
  listed in résumé, 77
  providing, 86
  for students, 103
Registered nurses, as knowledge
  workers, 18-19
Relocation, and retirement,
  142-143, 142b
Resource(s)
  for career planning, 51-58,
    52f-57f, 58b

Resource(s) *(Continued)*
  for entrepreneurs/intrepreneurs,
    126-129, 127f-128f
  Internet as, 58
  self-assessment of, 31-32,
    126-129
Résumé(s), 66-67
  chronological, 67, 69f-70f
  cover letter for, 78-80, 80f, 81f
  creation of, 73-77
  curriculum vitae (CV) compared,
    67, 68f
  do's and don'ts of, 78f
  electronic, 77-78, 79b
  functional, 71, 71f-73f, 77
  hybrid, 73, 74f-76f
  of students, 102-103
  types of, 67-73, 69f-70f, 71f-73f,
    74f-76f
Retirement, 138b
  healthy, 142-143
  lifestyle goals and, 46
  vision of, 140-143
  working after, 143
Retirement planning, 135-145
  process of, 137-144
  self-assessment in, 137-140
    of benefits of work, 137-137
    of financial status, 139
    of priorities, 138-139
    of readiness for retirement,
      140
    of skills and talents, 139
  for women, 136-137
Risk taking, in career action plan,
  45, 46b
Role enhancement goals, 46

**S**

Scanning, of environment, 7-8,
  12-21, 20f
  by entrepreneurs/intrepreneurs,
    123-124
  during retirement planning,
    137
  by students, 95
Self-actualization, 24-25
Self-assessment, 8, 22-33